Taking Over the Asylum

Also by Marian Barnes and Ric Bowl:

Sectioned: Social Services and the 1983 Mental Health Act (with Mike Fisher)

Also by Marian Barnes:

Care, Communities and Citizens

Women and Mental Health (with Norma Maple)

Taking Over the Asylum

Empowerment and Mental Health

Marian Barnes and Ric Bowl

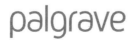

First published 2001 by
PALGRAVE
Houndmills, Basingstoke, Hampshire RG21 6XS and
175 Fifth Avenue, New York, N.Y. 10010
Companies and representatives throughout the world

PALGRAVE is the new global academic imprint of
St. Martin's Press LLC Scholarly and Reference Division and
Palgrave Publishers Ltd (formerly Macmillan Press Ltd).

ISBN 0–333–74091–2 paperback

This book is printed on paper suitable for recycling and made from fully managed and sustained forest sources.

A catalogue record for this book is available from the British Library.

Editing and origination by
Aardvark Editorial, Mendham, Suffolk

10 9 8 7 6 5 4 3 2 1
10 09 08 07 06 05 04 03 02 01

Printed in Malaysia

*To colleagues and friends in the
mental health users/survivors movement*

Contents

Preface   x

1   Mental health and empowerment   **1**
What is the problem?   1
Capacity, competence and rationality: the personal and
    interpersonal impacts of psychological distress   3
Managing madness   9
Can mental patients be citizens too?   13
Stigma, poverty and social exclusion   16
Dimensions and definitions of empowerment   17
Conclusion   24

2   From lunatics to survivors   **26**
Psychiatry and the welfare state   29
Proliferation and diversification   35
Developments within the state   41

3   Strategies for empowerment   **46**
Sites of action among mental health service users in
    the UK: implications and dilemmas   47
The policy context   56
Diverse objectives and strategies   63
Strategies and concepts of empowerment   66

4   Diversity, difference and empowerment   **68**
Crazy women   69
Women organising   75
Fighting mad   76
Ethnic difference and mental distress   80
Hospital admission and incidence rates of distress   80
Different colour, different treatment   82
Explanations of ethnic difference   83

Diagnosis, mis-diagnosis and racism   86
Black service users and the user movement   90

5   Changing lives and minds   **94**
Evaluating the impact of involvement strategies   94
Consultation and participation – therapeutic or
        democratic goals?   96
Consultation and participation within service
        establishments and their influence on service users   97
The effect of wider consultation and
        participation strategies   99
Fit for the purpose   102
Self-help, autonomous action and benefits
        for service users   105
The 'helper-therapy principle'   108
Joint working   112
Changing the professionals and the public   113

6   Changing the system   **117**
Surveys, focus groups and consultation exercises   118
Following through   120
Achievements in partnership   121
Advantages of independence   123
Resistance and representation   124
Conflicting demands, contrasting discourses   127
Different expectations and limited structures   130
The broader context   131

7   Social movements and social change   **134**
What are new social movements?   134
User and survivor movements as contemporary
        social movements   138
Contested identities   140
Making links   143
Social movements and social change strategies   144
Self-interest or social change?   148
Conclusion   152

8   Future prospects   **153**
      The evidence so far   153
      Rediscovering inequality and community   156
      Enabling participation   162
      Broader decision-making within service organisations   163
      Training and education   164
      Involvement strategies and movement goals   165

References   167

Index   182

Preface

In this book we explore what has been referred to earlier as 'Power in Strange Places' (Barker and Peck, 1987). In doing so, we have drawn on research by ourselves and others and on the accounts of people who have lived with mental health problems and of service users and survivors who have been active in a growing movement. Our aim is both to contribute to an understanding of the transformations that are taking place in the way in which organised groups of service users are giving voice to the experience of 'madness', and to recognise and value the action being pursued by such groups. We are 'academics' but also have 'attitude' – we do not write as people who are neutral about the value of such action, but as people who have tried in our own spheres to work as allies with service users and survivors.

Our research has been conducted in England and our prime focus is on the UK user movement. That movement itself, however, is increasingly part of a European and wider network of groups throughout the world. Much of the research which has been conducted in this area comes from North America. We draw on this and on other research and accounts from Australia, New Zealand and parts of Europe to consider both similarities and differences in the maturing movement of service users.

The structure of the book is as follows. In Chapter 1 we discuss the way in which ideology, policy and practice have contributed to the 'disempowerment' of people who have been diagnosed with mental illness. We relate this to the varied and contested concepts of empowerment which have been advanced. We do so to argue for and analyse changes in the relationship between the state and its citizens – in particular as that relationship is mediated through the provision of welfare.

Chapter 2 provides a brief history of attempts by 'lunatics' and 'survivors' to influence the way in which they are treated and concludes with an introduction to the contemporary context within which such objectives are being pursued. In Chapter 3 we explore the different strategies being adopted by user groups and the way these relate to 'official' policy for user involvement.

Chapter 4 highlights the diversity within the experiences of those diagnosed as mentally ill, focusing on the significance of gender and 'race' in constructing the experience of severe psychological distress and affecting responses to it.

Chapters 5 and 6 consider evidence relating to the impact of collective action on the part of service users/survivors. We address the impact of such action on those directly involved, and on policies and practices within mental health services. Chapter 7 broadens the perspective to consider user/survivor movements as examples of new social movements seeking wider social change, and in Chapter 8 we consider future prospects for the movement in the context of a new discourse of partnership within public services.

We would like to thank all those people involved in the user movement with whom we have worked – both for contributing to our understanding and to the research and teaching in which we are involved. This book is dedicated to you.

1

Mental health and empowerment

What is the problem?

People who are seriously disadvantaged in society rarely have single problems – they have multiple interlocking problems. They do not compete on a level playing field. They suffer a 'cycle of deprivation'. Empowerment must address all their problems together if it is to be meaningful. Poverty, poor housing and the nature of the social security system put a strain on relationships and lead to widespread demoralisation. Depending on the circumstances of individuals they can lead to physical and mental ill health, criminality, addiction and the persecution of individual or collective scapegoats: racism, sexism, picking on individuals who are 'different'. Disadvantaged people usually can only afford to live in areas where there is poor air quality, low car ownership but heavy traffic and other inferior environmental conditions – particularly those which pose a danger to children and thereby add to the stress of their parents. (Davey, 1999: 37)

In this paragraph Brian Davey, who works with Ecoworks, an environmental project led by users of mental health services, identifies the multiple dimensions of disempowerment and disadvantage which are often experienced by people with mental health problems. Davey argues that all these dimensions need to be addressed if empowerment is to be a reality. In this book we aim to explore these various dimensions of disempowerment and consider ways in which people who have experienced mental distress are seeking to empower themselves and to challenge perceptions of themselves as irrational and incompetent. We explore the personal impact of severe psychological distress, the interaction between people experiencing such distress and formal systems of health and welfare, and the experiences of people in their relationships with their families, the communities in which they live and society as a whole. We discuss the way in which official policy may serve to contribute to exclusion as well as seek to overcome it, and the way in which professional practices themselves may empower or oppress. We describe action being taken by those who use mental health services to empower themselves and to help policy makers and practitioners to work with those who have experienced mental health problems to develop more effective services.

In order to set the scene for what follows, this chapter has two purposes. The first is to consider why empowerment may be a particular 'problem' in the case of people who are identified as mentally disordered or who experience mental health problems. The second purpose is to look at the concept of empowerment itself. It is a word which has entered the discourse of public policy in general and welfare services in particular, but is used to mean very different things and at times appears to lack any real content. Before we can examine in more detail ways in which people experiencing severe psychological distress may become more empowered, we need to understand both the different contexts in which the notion of empowerment is applied as well as the contested nature of the concept.

But first a word about terminology of mental health and mental illness. Language is itself a site of struggle and one of the purposes of user or survivor movements is to reclaim the right to define and name their own experiences. Not all those active in mental health user movements would take sides with the anti-psychiatrists and reject the notion of 'mental illness', although some do consider the notion of 'illness' an inappropriate way of understanding their distress. Some reject the tag 'user', either because of an implication of active engagement with services which does not correspond to the experience of receiving services, or because of the connotation of drug misuse. 'Consumer' is a term associated with rational choice theory and the market ideology predominant in the 1980s and early 1990s in both the UK and USA. In the UK some user activists have accepted the term (although not necessarily the ideology with which it is associated), but others have adopted the term 'survivor': 'to portray a positive image of people in distress and people whose experience differs from, or who dissent from, society's norms' (http://www.inc.co.uk/~acorn/acorn/survivor.htm). In the USA, activists have distinguished between the identities of 'consumers', 'ex-patients' or 'survivors' on the basis of an acceptance or rejection of the medical model of mental illness (McLean, 1995).

One of our purposes in this book is to explore the variety of positions and strategies adopted by those concerned with the empowerment of people who have used mental health services. Thus we will use a variety of terms to describe and understand such action and the experiences to which it relates. We will use the term: 'severe psychological distress' to describe the nature of the experience of those living with mental health problems, and 'mental disorder' when we are explicitly referring to those considered to fall within the scope of the current Mental Health Act of England and Wales (in which 'mental disorder' refers to mental illness, personality disorder and severe mental impairment). At times we will also use the term 'madness' when this can be considered to be a useful description of the impact of distress and the way this is perceived by others. Where possible we will use the terms people themselves use to describe the groups or action with which they are engaged. Thus we will refer both to 'users' and 'survivors' when this is the way people describe themselves, and 'consumers' when this is the term used either by mental health workers or users to describe themselves or those they are working with.

Capacity, competence and rationality: the personal and interpersonal impacts of psychological distress

The impact of severe psychological distress can be profoundly debilitating at a personal level and highly disruptive of interpersonal relationships. The accounts of those who have been diagnosed as mentally ill are testimony to the way in which this may undermine a person's sense of self as well as their relationships with friends, family and strangers. This undermining of self is particularly acute when the responses of others conflict with self-perceptions. The experience of psychological distress and of receiving mental health services are hard to disentangle. Once someone attracts a psychiatric diagnosis they often find themselves subject to others' decision making and others' definitions of their needs and problems – even when they are not subject to compulsory admission to hospital and the others are friends as well as mental health professionals. These responses become intermingled with the impact of the distress itself. Kate Millett describes this in her account of her experience of being diagnosed as suffering from manic depression and being subject to unwelcome interventions from both professionals and friends as a result:

> This is an account of a journey into that nightmare state ascribed to madness: that social condition, that experience of being cast out and confined. ...Some of us survive it intact, others only partially survive, debilitated by the harm

done to us: the temptations of complicity, of the career of 'patient', the pressures towards capitulation. (Millett, 1991: 11)

Similarly Judi Chamberlin records the way in which the help she hoped to receive from psychiatric services when she was experiencing considerable distress in fact undermined her sense of herself as someone who was capable of controlling her own life:

> Eleven years ago, I spent about five months as a patient in six mental hospitals. The experience totally demoralised me. I had never thought of myself as a particularly strong person, but after hospitalisation, I was convinced of my own worthlessness... For years I feared that any stress, any difficulty would lead to my total collapse. (Chamberlin, 1988: 5)

While personal accounts indicate that mental health services can exacerbate the disabling effect of psychological distress, this is not to deny the impact of the distress itself. Severe psychological distress can be the source of experiences which in themselves can be frightening, exhilarating, or profoundly anxiety provoking. Linda Hart, herself a nurse who once worked in the psychiatric hospital to which she was later admitted, describes the experience of living with madness which can threaten survival itself:

> My father is having fun with me. Threatening to take over the bit of my mind that functions. He's stopped directing various suicide scenarios. He can claim my psyche perhaps more easily. There are dangers everywhere here because it's so unreal. To tip over the last threads could happen so effortlessly because I'm so tired of it all. Get my head down. Get discharged. Get home and die. I'm plausible enough to make them think I'm well. (Hart, 1995: 15)

In addition to expressing the destructive impact of severe psychological distress, Hart's account suggests the protective role that mental health services may play – even when that role is unwelcome at the time. It is important to recognise that there *are* times when uninvited interventions may, in the long run, be capable of creating the conditions in which empowerment is possible and a failure to act on the part of mental health workers is the most destructive response. Users of mental health services who have been subject to compulsory hospital admission do not always reject the necessity for this (for example Campbell, 1998). This is one of the many aspects of the complexity of the notion of empowerment in the context of experiences of psychological distress to which we will return during the course of this book.

Perhaps the most destructive of all experiences of severe psychological distress is that of dementia. While it is very hard to access directly the experience of those who have dementia, observation of its impact has sometimes suggested a trickling away or fragmentation of the person. Those who live with someone with dementia describe an experience of being bereaved before death because the person has effectively, 'gone', even though they are still there physically. One attempt to enter into the mind of someone with dementia is described in Michael Ignatieff's novel *Scar Tissue* where he draws on his own observations of his mother to describe the impact of dementia both on the woman concerned and on those close to her. Bernlef (1988) similarly tries to enter into the mind of a man as dementia spreads through him and he approaches death. As the fragmentation process develops, the text becomes increasingly broken up – words and phrases no longer form sentences and one follows the other without apparent continuity. It is notable that some of the most effective means of capturing and seeking to understand the experience of dementia has been through the use of literary forms. While the narratives of people with dementia may appear to lack logical coherence, they have their own logic which may be more effectively expressed through the rhythms of poetic cadences than through everyday prose narratives (Killick, 1998). Killick uses his experiences as a poet to edit the words of people with dementia in order to 'pare away what I judge to be inessential, leaving the primary material standing clear' (ibid.: 14) This process can demonstrate how people with dementia may be hanging on to their own sense of identity, their own empowerment even, but that such identity can be inaccessible to the majority of those without insight into the utterances of the speakers.

One problem for people experiencing psychological distress and for those close to them is the huge variation in mood and behaviour that can result. Such unpredictability can make relationships difficult and lead to relationship breakdown. There is an ambiguous relationship between family life and mental health. While men are more likely to be admitted to psychiatric hospitals if they are single, the majority of women admitted are married (Barnes and Maple, 1992), although levels of psychosis and neurosis within community populations have been found to be lower among married women than among single women (Nazroo, 1997). Emotional relationships within families have been cited as contributory factors in psychological distress (Leff and Vaughan, 1985), but there is also evidence of people experiencing psychological distress making contributions to family wellbeing and being supported by their families in achieving increased community participation (Greenberg *et al.*,1994). Living with a relative experiencing severe psychological distress can be a source of considerable difficulty for parents, partners and other family members. The wishes of those experiencing severe psychological distress and their families about their treatment and about the way in which they want to live their lives can often be a matter of conflict (Lefley, 1996).

Mental illness may involve experiences which are hard to make sense of and can cause fear and confusion, making it very difficult for people to get on with their daily lives:

> I was so paranoid. I mean I used to duck and dive in hedges, you know. I used to think the IRA were after me, or if there was a murder on the television, I thought the murderer was following me, and every time the police caught somebody I used to feel relieved for a little while. (Ritchie *et al.*, 1988: 5)

This is one reason for the widespread fear of madness: the sense of unpredictability, lack of control and the apparent lack of rationality in behaviour. This fear can lead to exclusion and rejection which in turn can result in people seeking to hide their distress and thus not seek help.

While psychological distress may be a temporary or intermittent experience, it can come to define the whole self. Ben, a young man with a diagnosis of schizophrenia, talked of the way in which that diagnosis defines him in a way that could not happen if he suffered from a physical condition:

> I like to show that even though I have the illness, I can function as a person. If I had a broken leg, I wouldn't say 'I am a broken leg'. In the same way, we shouldn't say 'I am a schizophrenic...' I might limp or something, but it shouldn't define your life... I don't want to be a schizophrenic 'doing well': 'Isn't he good even though he's had a mental illness?' I just want my illness to be forgotten about. I'm not proud of it, its a bloody nuisance. I hate being called a schizophrenic. (quoted in Barham and Barnes, 1999: 140)

Nevertheless, once having received a diagnosis and having experienced the impact of psychological distress, it can be hard to be as confident that you have been 'cured' as it is in the case of a physical illness. Thus any sense of 'recovery' is fragile and people who have used mental health services often cannot confidently describe themselves as 'ex-users'. In a research interview an activist in a user group said to us: 'You never know when you stop being a user'. The effects of psychological distress remain for a long time. And unlike a spent criminal conviction, a record as a psychiatric patient can affect people's prospects throughout their lives and consequently both their social relationships and economic circumstances.

Severe psychological distress can affect anyone, regardless of age, social class, ethnicity or gender. But the experience is not equally distributed, nor is the nature of the experience the same across all social groups. Many women who end up using mental health services have experienced sexual or physical abuse. For some, entering hospital does not mean moving to a place of safety and asylum but entering another environment in which they are at risk – from both staff and fellow patients (Wood and Copperman, 1996). Similarly, for black people the experience of psychological distress cannot be separated from experiences of racism, both within the mental health system and beyond. In Chapter 4 we focus specifically on the experiences of women and of black people as users of services and as activists within the user movement. But the general point to make here is that the disempowering impact of distress may be related to other experiences of exclusion and oppression and that action to empower users of mental health services must recognise and respond to the multiple dimensions of disempowerment involved.

Closely associated with the impact of severe psychological distress on the person themselves, and in turn on their relationships with others and the world around them, are the notions of irrationality and incompetence. Madness is understood as a loss of reason. The term 'mental disorder' reflects the perception that both disordered thinking and disordered behaviour provide the evidence for the existence of a mental illness. Those suffering from mental illness are often described as 'lacking insight' into their condition. The nature of their condition is seen to be such that it prevents them from understanding that there is anything wrong with them. They may also be considered to be incapable of taking control over their own lives and thus 'for their own good' need to be subject to compulsory powers.

Doyal and Gough (1991) define 'autonomy' as one of the basic and universal human needs. Individual autonomy is affected by three variables: the level of understanding a person has about herself, her culture and what is expected of her within it, her psychological capacity to formulate options for herself, and the objective opportunities there are for her to act accordingly. 'Mental illness' is perceived as a factor which severely impairs autonomy, leading, in some instances to action being taken to reduce the objective opportunities for individuals so identified to act autonomously (for example, when people are compulsorily detained under the Mental Health Act). In some instances those experiencing severe psychological distress themselves report 'reduced psychological capacity'. People may become highly disturbed or highly depressed and find it difficult to pursue a course of action that they might wish. This is one reason why advocacy has been developed as a model to enable people to have their voices heard.

Doyal and Gough recognise the cultural specificity of many behaviours which might be taken as indication of 'non-rational' responses to events or circumstance. However, they suggest that there are factors necessary to the existence of minimal levels of autonomy, regardless of cultural context:

(a) that actors have the intellectual capacity to formulate aims and beliefs common to a form of life;
(b) that actors have enough confidence to want to act and thus to participate in a form of life;
(c) that actors sometimes actually do so, consistently formulating aims and beliefs and communicating with others about them;
(d) that actors perceive their actions as having been done by them and not by someone else;
(e) that actors are able to understand the empirical constraints on the success of their actions;
(f) that actors are capable of taking responsibility for what they do (ibid.: 63).

Individual judgements about the level of autonomy of any particular individual at any particular time are affected by variables such as gender and 'race' as well as by the professional and epistemological frameworks within which individuals are making such judgements (Allen, 1987; Busfield, 1996). The capacity to exercise agency is not constant and can be enhanced or reduced by the actions and responses of others. Both lay and professional constructions of 'mental illness' associate this with irrationality and reduced levels of autonomy in a way which does not apply to physical illness. If, by definition, someone experiencing severe psychological distress is perceived as having impaired autonomy then this has important implications for their level of empowerment – both because of the impact this can have on perceptions of self, and because this can lead to actions which reduce objective opportunities to exercise autonomy.

We have now reached the point at which we need to turn to the way in which public policies have developed to respond to the care, treatment and management of people experiencing severe psychological distress. These polices and practices also serve to define the terrain within which any discussion of the potential 'empowerment' of people experiencing distress must be considered.

Managing madness

A historical and comparative analysis of the way in which 'the mentally disordered' are 'managed' within society illustrates the way in which social policies and professional practices serve to reflect different understandings of what mental disorders or illnesses are (Fernando, 1991; Prior, 1993). While it is necessary to understand the way in which psychological distress can affect the person themselves and those with whom they live their lives, we have already seen how this cannot be disentangled from the response people receive from both lay and professional people. This reflects the dominant discourse within which mental illness is defined and negotiated. In a society in which the scientific rationality of enlightenment thinking provides the key point of reference, the irrationality of the insane presents a profound threat to social order as well as to personal integrity.

The emergence in the late nineteenth century of a particular category of medical specialists who claimed the treatment of the insane as their territory was part of a broader movement through which the medical profession gained hegemonic control over many areas of knowledge and experience which had not previously been defined as issues of illnesses or treatment (Ehrenreich and English, 1979; Foucault, 1980; Turner, 1995). Foucault has argued that the transformation of medicine in the nineteenth century involved a shift from a perception of medicine as assistance, to an emphasis on the role of medicine as an apparatus of power to ensure good health and thus an economically productive population. In his book *Madness and Civilization* he argues that the exercise of control in relation to the 'unreason' represented by mental illness operates through the suppression of irrationality by rational scientific knowledge. Madness itself is suppressed by being designated as mental illness, to be dealt with by the man of science who has delegated authority to use the power of abstract reason to communicate between the mad man and society (Foucault, 1965).

The tensions between the social control and care and treatment roles of psychiatry have been a continuing source of controversy within the history of mental health services. As what had earlier been described as madness, delirium, folly, or melancholy, became defined in terms of illness or disease, a range of clinical professions moved in to offer their explanations of causes and hence treatment responses (Prior, 1993). Throughout the twentieth century the field became increasingly crowded. Psychiatrists, psychologists, psychoanalysts, psychotherapists, social workers and psychiatric nurses offer their own particular perspectives on the human experience defined as mental illness and on how this should be treated – not only in the interests of the 'sufferer', but also in order to protect the rest of society. Professional disputes over the ownership of psychological distress have become more evident as the terrain has become more crowded (Figert, 1996; Pilgrim, 1997a). As Figert in particular has demonstrated in her analysis of the dispute over whether pre-menstrual syndrome should be included as a psychiatric diagnosis (see Chapter 4), the voices of those who are subject to such professional disputes are often comparatively uninfluential as professional power blocks encounter each other, each claiming the legitimacy of their particular knowledge and authority.

It is not only within the sphere of the social history of medicine and related professions that we need to look to understand the way in which social policies relating to the care and treatment of mentally disordered people have developed. Richard Warner (1994) traces the links between the treatment of people with a diagnosis of schizophrenia and the developing political economies of western societies. Arguing the need for a materialist theoretical approach to the study of schizophrenia Warner claims:

> A materialist research strategy, for example, allows us to generate the hypothesis that social attitudes towards the insane partly reflect the usefulness of the psychotic person in the productive process; that psychiatric ideology is influenced by economic conditions; that the course of schizophrenia is influenced by class status, sex roles and labor dynamics; or that variations in the occurrence of the illness may reflect differences in the circumstances of different classes and castes under different modes of subsistence and production. (ibid.: xi)

The nature of work and way in which it is organised have affected the extent to which people experiencing psychological distress have been seen to be capable of having a role to play within social and economic systems. As capitalist economies grew more demanding of consistent discipline among workers, the less formalised and localised work opportunities which had been available to those who might be somewhat erratic in their labour started to disappear. The need to separate out those who not only were seen to be unable to make an efficient contribution to economic development, but who were also in danger of tainting the rest led to policies of segregation.

Segregating the sane from the insane in institutions away from the urban centres in which the population was increasingly being concentrated was intended to have therapeutic effects for those incarcerated, as well as to be protective of the normal 'population'. They would no longer be threatened by the moral taint or physical threat offered by the mad (Prior, 1993). This dual function of therapy and segregation has been recognised by those who have questioned the inevitability of the progress represented by the move at the end of the twentieth century to close the asylums and move those previously resident within them back into the communities from which they had been segregated for so long:

> A rather less sanguine account of what policies of deinstitutionalisation actually amount to suggests, as we have seen, that they have by and large been powered by more expedient motives. On this reading, far from returning home after a long period of exile, many people with mental illness are being ejected from the refuges which over a long period had protected them from the brunt of market forces and told to go and shift for themselves as best they can. On this view, all the talk about providing new opportunities for individuals to flourish and to determine their own lives is just a rhetorical disguise worn by those governmental agencies who are intent on dumping a group of people whom it has become too costly to maintain in the old welfare style. (Barham, 1992: 99)

Whatever the major engine driving the closure of long-stay psychiatric hospitals (and whatever the potential and indeed actual benefits of the asylum and facilities offered by long-stay hospitals) one important reason for closure was the evidence of dehumanisation and abuse, as well as of their simple lack of capacity to respond to the individual needs of all those contained within them. By the end of the 1990s the closure process had led to a major shift in the way in which mental health services were being provided. There have been many versions of community care policy and a real understanding of the notion of 'community' has been absent from most official versions (Barnes, 1997). It has been argued that it is not enough for people formerly resident in long-stay institutions to be 'in the community', but that it is also necessary for them to have a valued role within that community (Ramon, 1991). Research which followed up people who had been discharged from long-stay psychiatric hospitals identified improved social behaviour, everyday living skills and freedom from restrictions experienced by the former patients, but also the fact that public attitudes formed a barrier to increased social participation (Leff, 1997).

If there is now a fairly widespread belief that long-term geographical segregation of people experiencing psychological distress is only justified in cases where there is evidence of actual harm having been done by or to the mentally disordered person, there is still a view that they should be subject to a level of control and supervision which most of the population would regard as a wholly unjustifiable constraint on their own autonomy. The UK Royal College of Psychiatrists campaigned for an amendment to the 1983 Mental Health Act to introduce a community treatment or community supervision order. This received partial support in December 1993 when the Department of Health announced a requirement on all health authorities to establish and maintain supervision registers identifying those people diagnosed with a mental illness who were also considered to be a significant risk to themselves or others. The argument for this was based in part on experience of legislation providing for community treatment in other countries. For example, in Victoria (Australia) the 1986 Mental Health Act includes such a provision and similar proposals were made to introduce such an order in New South Wales. The guidance from the NHS Executive (1994) relating to the establishment of supervision registers and supervised discharge stated:

> Those taking individual decisions about discharge have a fundamental duty to consider both the safety of the patient and the protection of other people. No patient should be discharged from hospital unless and until those taking the decisions are satisfied that he or she can live safely in the community, and that proper treatment, supervision, support and care are available. (para 2, p. 1)

This reluctance to adopt the same perspective on patient autonomy in the case of people diagnosed with mental illness as defined by both law and practice relating to people with a physical illness has continued to affect mental health policy. 'Modernising Mental Health Services' a government White Paper published in 1998 identified safety as the first principle on which services should be based: 'services should be safe, *to protect the public* and provide effective care for those with mental illness at the time they need it' (our italics). The document announces that 'care in the community has failed' and (in spite of the establishment of supervision registers) so too has there been a failure to ensure continuity of care after discharge from hospital. The proposed remedies for these failures included investment to provide more beds and a rigorous performance management framework. Assertive outreach was hailed as the mains of engaging people who 'are typically hard to engage because of their negative experiences of statutory services' (para 4.21). This approach involves regular, intensive contact with people experiencing psychological distress who, although not subject to compulsory orders, can find themselves on the receiving end of intervention concerned not only with compliance with medication, but also with where they live and how they spend their time. Evidence suggests that assertive outreach results in fewer emergency admissions and a reduction in symptoms, but this approach is further evidence of a policy based on a perception of people diagnosed as mentally ill needing to be 'taken charge of' for their own good.

This perception of people experiencing psychological distress as having impaired autonomy also affects their status as citizens.

Can mental patients be citizens too?

The status of 'citizen' is a disputed one in the UK because of the absence of a written constitution and the fact that, formally, the British people are subjects of the crown. The discourse of citizenship is often regarded as 'foreign' and few readily identify themselves as citizens. Nevertheless, concepts of justice and fair treatment are familiar and common in lay discourse suggesting that there are assumptions about the rights assumed to attach to community membership, irrespective of formal rights enshrined in a constitution. The significance of those rights is perhaps more evident to those whose experience is of being deprived of them. The disabled people's movement has adopted an explicit civil rights perspective and, while this is less explicit among mental health user movements, achieving fair and just treatment is a key underpinning of the objectives of user and survivor movements (Barnes and Shardlow, 1996; Campbell and Oliver, 1996).

A starting point for most contemporary analyses of citizenship within liberal western societies is that of Marshall (1950) who defined citizenship rights as comprising:

- legal or civil rights which enable the individual to participate freely in the life of the community. These include property and contractual rights; rights to freedom of thought, freedom of speech, religious practice, assembly and association;

- political rights which entitle the citizen to participate in the government of the community: the right to vote and to hold political office;

- social and economic rights to the circumstances which enable the individual to participate in the general wellbeing of the community. They include rights to health care, education and welfare.

A designation of mental incapacity can result in certain formal exclusions from the civil rights associated with citizenship (Law Commission, 1995). For example, if a judge considers a person to be incapable of managing their property or affairs due to mental incapacity the Court of Protection can be invoked to take over the administration of their financial and other affairs. Similarly, contracts entered into by those subsequently considered to be mentally incapacitated at the time may be declared invalid. While such measures are designed to protect people from exploitation, they also represent a constraint on basic citizenship rights.

The potential for compulsory detention and for medical treatment administered without consent also represent constraints on the freedoms associated with the civil rights of citizenship. Treatment without consent for physical conditions can only be applied in emergency conditions when waiting to obtain consent could result in death (for example when people are unconscious following a road traffic accident). While only a minority of people with mental health problems are subject to the provisions of the Mental Health Act, the possibility and fear of 'sectioning' has a much wider impact on people's sense of their identity as autonomous citizens. Evidence of an increase in the proportion of people entering hospital compulsorily (MHAC, 1995) and the extension of the controlling powers of mental health legislation through the introduction of supervised discharge procedures discussed above represent constraints on citizenship rights of an increasing number of people considered mental disordered.

Political rights have also been subject to constraint. While detention in a psychiatric hospital should not automatically result in debarring people from voting, the residence requirement for voting registration has been used effectively to exclude detained patients from being able to exercise their right to vote. In practice, people who have spent long periods in psychiatric hospitals have been denied the opportunity to vote. This has been the subject of a campaign led by MIND in the UK which also involved a challenge to the European Court (MIND, 1997).

But it is perhaps in the area of social and economic rights that the constraints on the citizenship of substantial number of people experiencing severe psychological distress is most evident. A renewal of interest in the notion of citizenship recognises that it is not only a political but also a sociological concept (for example van Steenbergen, 1994). Citizenship is not only a status to which are attached a series of actual or assumed rights, but a practice through which individuals relate to their communities and to the state (Prior *et al.*, 1995). In considering the impact of psychological distress we should be thinking not only about formal constraints on citizenship rights, but how this experience may interfere with their capacity to 'practise as citizens'.

Prior *et al.* locate the practice of citizenship within the tripartite relationship between the individual, state and civil society. Citizens are active participants in a 'network of rights and obligations, freedoms and restrictions, which is constantly being renegotiated and which thereby continually redefines the spheres of actions, of individuals, state and civil society' (ibid.: 20–1). Ranson *et al.* (1995) locate citizenship as a practice in which people are active agents in defining and creating a civil society which recognises and includes difference. Similarly Lister emphasises the connections between citizenship, agency and autonomy: 'Citizenship as participation represents an expression of human agency in the political arena, broadly defined; citizenship as rights enables people to act as agents' (Lister, 1997: 36). Thus citizenship is not solely a question of the rights and obligations attached to membership of a political community, but also of the extent to which space is provided for people to contribute to the creation of their social world. In terms of the relationship between the individual and state this can mean, in practice, the extent to which people are able to contribute to the creation of public services which are often the form through which this relationship is mediated. In the sphere of civil society it can refer, for example, to the potential for people who have experienced psychological distress to use the visual arts or media to create images of madness or disability which can challenge stereotypes, as well as to create their own organisations which can support fellow sufferers or provide alternative forms of 'service'.

This analysis is relevant to the consideration of ways in which people who have experienced mental health problems might both express and be considered to occupy the status of 'citizen'. We will return to this as we discuss the way in which collective organisation among people who have experienced severe psychological distress has made a significant contribution to their empowerment.

Stigma, poverty and social exclusion

The concept of autonomy embraces not only the psychological capacity to act, but also the objective opportunities to act. Such opportunities can be constrained by poverty as well as by the exclusionary attitudes of others. Our notions of citizenship are related to those of inclusion or exclusion. Indeed the multilayered concept of social exclusion can be taken to refer to the varied routes and mechanisms by which people come to be regarded as effectively occupying a position of 'non-citizen' for all practical purposes. If a citizen is not only a rights bearer but also someone who contributes to the creation of the social world, then those who are regarded as incompetent to take decisions on their own behalf and who are considered to need the interventions of welfare agencies 'for their own good' might be considered to stand outside the world of active citizenship. At a more practical level, if the day-to-day struggle for survival, not only in emotional terms, but also in material terms, takes up all your energy, to what extent can you be considered to be in a position to contribute to 'creating the social world?'

Research has demonstrated the practical impact of stigma experienced by people diagnosed with a mental illness. For example a survey conducted by MIND revealed that 34 per cent of those responding said they had been dismissed or forced to resign from their jobs, 47 per cent said they had been abused or harassed in public, 26 per cent were forced to move home as a result of harassment, 25 per cent had been turned down by insurance or finance companies (Read and Baker, 1996). People with mental health problems have the highest rate of unemployment among disabled people – 38 per cent compared with 21 per cent overall among disabled people (Lunt and Thornton, 1996).

Others have also documented not only the absolute poverty in which many people with severe psychological distress live their lives, but also the debilitating effects of the struggle to deal with the complexities of the welfare system (Davis and Betteridge, 1997; Hogman and Chapman,

1998). The personal impact of poverty and unemployment, and the uncertainty caused by social security changes can further exacerbate the impact of distress itself:

> I was now pushed into a situation while I was at [bed and breakfast hotel] where I was in absolute poverty. I didn't even have enough to live on. I had to go back to my parents with my hands out... after I'd supposedly broken away and become independent and learned how to manage for myself. It wasn't very dignifying. (male, 20s, now living in group home) (quoted in Ritchie *et al.*, 1988: 8)

> Due to the reviews in state benefits my illness has become unbearable. I have had increased medication to calm me down: that is, Diazepam, Chlorpromazine after much reassurance from doctors, family and friends everything will be OK and so on. I do not think that anyone that does not suffer from this or any type of mental illness knows exactly the effects it's having on our state of mind. Everyday living is bad enough with the problems of mental illness without having this added worry. (quoted in Hogman and Chapman, 1998: 2)

The practical constraints on the lives of people who might formerly have been mental patients but who are now 'in the community' has led Peter Barham to suggest: 'Release from the stigmatizing discourse of psychiatry may not entail much more than the freedom to be picked up in the stigmatizing discourse of poverty.' (Barham, 1992: 105).

Dimensions and definitions of empowerment

The preceding analysis has identified what we might consider the 'dimensions of disempowerment' within the lives of people living with severe psychological distress. It has highlighted the negative impact of such distress and of the position people with a diagnosis of mental illness can find themselves in: in their interpersonal relationships, in their relationships with the mental health service system and in their position as citizens within the communities in which they live. However, this picture of personal distress and of social exclusion is far from being the whole story and as this book progresses we will explore just why it would be wrong to regard people with psychological distress as passive victims of their illnesses or of the social circumstances in which they find themselves.

But it is important to understand the different dimensions of *disempowerment* in order to understand the nature of the strategies necessary to promote empowerment. In the remainder of this chapter we consider the way in which *empowerment* has been conceptualised by those expressing commitment to policies and practices intended to empower users of mental health services as well as others who are on the receiving end of the sometimes paternalistic, other times directly controlling powers of an increasingly risk-averse welfare state.

The term 'empowerment' has been used promiscuously to refer to a wide range of very different processes and practices. Thinking on empowerment has been developed within academic disciplines of sociology, social policy, psychology and politics, while those engaged in practical action in social work, community development, nursing and other areas of social welfare and community action have also developed their own definitions and their own conclusions about 'empowering practice' (for example Braye and Preston-Shoot 1995; Parsloe, 1996; Pithouse and Williamson, 1997). Researchers have recognised the need to develop new research practice which reflects the values of empowerment (for example Fetterman *et al.*, 1996; Barnes and Mercer, 1997; Barnes and Warren, 1999). There have also been attempts by researchers to develop scales to measure empowerment. For example, Rogers *et al.* (1997) identified five factors which define personal constructs of empowerment according to 'consumers' of mental health services. The criteria they suggested needed to be applied to measure empowerment were: self-efficacy–self-esteem, power–powerlessness, community activism, righteous anger, and optimism–control over the future. These criteria reflect both psychological and political dimensions of the concept.

In the context of social policy and health and social care practice, empowerment is often conceptualised in terms of a shift in the nature of the relationship between those who provide and those who receive services. A typical example comes from Parsloe in her introduction to a collection of contributions entitled *Pathways to Empowerment*:

> No definitive definition of empowerment is offered here because the concept is still evolving and it means different things to different people. It is used to refer to users of social services having greater control over the services they receive and here is concerned with the individual service level. It can also refer to a more general level of planning for services at the local, regional or national level when service users are involved in advising, and less frequently in deciding on the services to be provided. It may be seen as a way to reduce

professional power or a plot used cynically by professionals to protect their status and power. Its purpose may be to promote the personal growth of those empowered, to raise the quality and appropriateness of social services or to give the disadvantaged members of society some influence which may lead to their attaining greater political power. (Parsloe, 1996: xvii)

In her contribution on the topic of empowerment in social work practice in the same collection, Parsloe identifies the ambiguity inherent in the notion that 'clients' might be empowered by social workers:

It [empowerment] is a most unfortunate word for social work to have adopted because it can well be argued that the very idea that one person, a social worker, can empower another, a client, runs counter to the whole idea of greater equality of power on which the concept supposedly depends. (ibid.: 6)

Nevertheless, the development of practices which have the potential to contribute to 'clients' *becoming empowered* became a feature of social work and other social care practices during the 1990s. In the context of the professional practice of workers within the mental health system the issue is, first, how can therapeutic relationships be negotiated to achieve shared understandings and objectives within a context in which the professional has considerably more objective power than the user? Second, can such relationships enable 'clients' to empower themselves in other aspects of their lives? We will consider the potential of such practices to contribute to the empowerment of people living with psychological distress in Chapter 8.

There is some difference of view about whether giving service users more control over the services they receive means that welfare professionals inevitably lose power, or whether a practice which can contribute to user empowerment can be experienced as not 'taking something away' from the professional concerned. The difference is rooted in views as to whether there is an absolute amount of power which might be redistributed but which cannot be increased (the 'zero sum' view), or whether power can increase and thus different stakeholders may gain (albeit in different ways) from increasing the power of those formerly occupying powerless positions.

A zero sum view of power would suggest that empowering a previously powerless individual or group requires *disempowering* (at least to some degree) those who already hold power. Power passes from one place to another. In practical terms this might mean that whereas decisions about, for example, the distribution of resources were previously taken by a group of health service commissioners, the power to make these decisions is shifted to a group of health service users. Professionals lose the power of decision making by delegating this elsewhere. In practice, within public services subject to rules of accountability, there is a limit to the extent that power, or more appropriately 'authority' to determine how public money is spent can be delegated. Thus while it is possible to point to numerous examples of mechanisms to consult with or work with service users to determine priorities for service development, service design and provision, there are far fewer examples of delegated power being given to service users. In those cases where there has been such delegation this has often been through contracting processes which have their own rules governing accountability.

But taking power over people is rather different from taking power over the use of resources. Exercising power over people involves the use of explicit or implicit coercion. The compulsory admission to hospital of people identified as mentally disordered is one example of explicit coercive power. The internalisation of messages that you are not capable of taking decisions in your own best interests can be understood as an implicit use of coercive power. If people experiencing severe psychological distress are repeatedly told that they 'have no insight into their condition', that they are incapable of making rational choices about what is in their best interests, then they may come to believe that they have no capacity to control what happens to them and thus internalise their own powerlessness.

This example demonstrates that the notion of empowerment as a process which somehow reverses the existing exercise of power over people may not be helpful. While people who have been diagnosed with a mental illness may wish to exercise more control over whether or not they receive mental health care and treatment, it is unlikely that most would want to exercise power over individual mental health professionals. In this context notions of partnership, shared decision making, or negotiation may be a more appropriate way of conceptualising the nature of the relationship being sought. A model of partnership practice which enables the knowledge and insights of both user and professional to be drawn on in developing problem-solving strategies not only has the potential to produce better outcomes for the user, it can also provide learning opportunities for professional actors to develop better practice (Marsh and Fisher, 1992). Both user and professional can benefit as a result.

However, notions of partnership or shared decision making may be just as complex as notions of empowerment. This is relevant to understanding the micro-politics of interactions taking place in the context of initiatives apparently intended to 'empower' service users by enabling them to be present in consultation and sometimes decision-making forums. Where opportunities for consultation or participation are determined by public agencies they operate within a particular institutional context which shapes the rules of the game within which users can take part. Critiques of deliberative democracy have suggested that this is based in liberal notions which ignore both cultural differences and the different social positions of those the practice seeks to engage (for example Young, 1996). Kathryn Church (1996) has analysed both users' and professionals' experiences of a process which was intended to 'empower' users in the context of consultation over mental health legislation in Canada. Her analysis illustrates the way in which power was embedded within the rules governing the processes through which user input was sought. In particular she considers the way in which the survivor stories told within these processes and the emotionality of the survivors' presentational styles were constructed as 'bad manners' and non-rational contributions. Their legitimacy in the decision-making process was thus contested by the professional members of the working party. Power is exercised not only by direct acts of coercion, but also in the context of apparently sympathetic initiatives to build closer relations with users. We discuss the processes involved as users of mental health services have sought to develop new relationships with service providers in Chapters 3 and 6.

A rather different view of empowerment is that it should be understood as a process in which people develop 'power to' take decisions, take actions, make choices, or work with others which they were previously unable to do. It is a conception which is based in notions of agency rather than structure. It is also a conception which does not involve coercive power to make people do things, but rather a generative process which increases the capacity to act and to enable others to do so. It can operate at both individual and collective levels, but often is maximised through acting with others. This creates new possibilities for action as well as supporting the development of shared understandings of sources of oppression resulting from coercive power being exercised over people. Generative power does not require the passage of power from one location to another, but nor can it be granted to people.

Empowerment, then, is not restricted to the achievement of the 'power over' form of power, but can also involve the development of power to, with and from within. These kinds of power are not finite; indeed, one might argue that the more they are exercised the more power can grow. (Rowlands, 1998: 15)

Anderson, J. (1996) takes a similar position and also identifies the way in which those who have been marginalised or oppressed can exercise power through resistance:

As Janeway points out, even the weak are not without power: they have the power to disbelieve; the power to come together as a group to act towards common goals; and they have the power to organise for action. So resistance to oppressive structures can be seen as an exercise of power, with disempowerment arising from a lack of resistance: 'the succumbing to conditions as they are or appear to be'.

Resistance can be achieved through subversion. In the context of an analysis of community responses to AIDS, Altman argues that subversion operating in the sphere of knowledge is particularly significant within areas of social life dominated by scientific knowledge and professional power:

Real 'development'... is inherently subversive. It is particularly subversive when, as with AIDS, it requires the recognition and empowerment of people who are often marginalized – sex workers, gay men, injecting drug users and, more broadly, women, children and the poor. Above all the search to empower those with AIDS themselves becomes, as we shall see, subversive of some of the most dominant discourses of power in the modern world, those based on medical and scientific authority and expertise. (Altman, 1994: 11)

Strategies emphasising the subversive power of different forms of knowledge reflect Foucault's analysis of the way in which dominant discourses act as a means through which power is exercised. We discuss the significance of this in the context of action among mental health service users in Chapter 7.

It should be clear by now that neither the concept of empowerment, nor effective strategies through which people experiencing psychological distress might become empowered, can be defined solely by changes in their relationships with mental health services. It is significant that, while in her introductory essay quoted above, Parsloe (1996) starts from ways in which people can come to exert more control over services (both individually and collectively), she immediately finds herself having to stray outside this relationship to try to capture what empowerment is all about. Through exercising more control over services, Parsloe speculates that empowerment may contribute both to personal growth and increased political power. Similarly, drawing on an analysis of the experience of older people seeking to influence health and social care services, Barnes and Walker (1996) have defined eight 'Principles of empowerment' which also reflect the wider context within which empowerment must be achieved.

Davey (quoted at the opening of this chapter) has distinguished 'reactive' from 'proactive' empowerment. Reactive empowerment refers to the situation in which people may find themselves in terms of their relationships with service systems where action is necessary to respond to unhelpful or disempowering action by service providers. Advocacy may be necessary to ensure that people's views are represented in reaction to a negative aspect of the system. Proactive empowerment involves the articulation of needs and wishes in ways which are not defined by nor dependant on the actions of those working within the mental health (or any other) system. This may lead to action to set up services outside the system, or to develop forms of organisation which are based round aspects of people's lives with which mainstream mental health services may have little concern. Throughout this book we will consider practical examples of action based in notions of both reactive and proactive empowerment.

There are three further issues which we will be exploring during the course of this book to which we also need to make reference in this introductory analysis of the notion of empowerment. The first concerns the relationship between user empowerment and carer empowerment. The identification of carers as a distinct group with legitimate interests to be represented within the health and social care system has, in some instances, led to conflict between carers and service users. In the UK and the USA some 'consumer' or advocacy groups are effectively carers' groups rather than groups controlled by people experiencing severe psychological distress themselves and the position they take often reflects a very different point of view from that of users themselves (see for example Lefley, 1996). People who have been diagnosed as mentally ill may receive considerable support from their families, but they can also experience family relationships as a source of tension and dispute. The significance of family life and family relationships in the context of initiatives which seek the empowerment of people who receive social care services has been considered in relation to children at risk (Boushel and Farmer, 1996) and people with learning difficulties (Barnes, 1997). We will consider the way in which organised groups of carers are claiming their own rights to empowerment and reflect on the implications of this for relationships between people experiencing severe psychological distress and family members in Chapter 2.

The second issue of particular relevance to a consideration of empowerment and mental health is the association between empowerment and health. Community development for health is based on a belief that to become healthy, both individuals and communities need to become empowered. Empowerment is seen as a precondition for enabling people to increase control over and improve their health (Hancock, 1993). We will consider what evidence there is to support this claim in the context of mental health in Chapter 5.

Finally, we need to consider the extent to which any action from within service systems or from among those defined as users of mental health services can address the structural dimensions of inequality and disempowerment to which we have referred earlier in this chapter. One view of empowerment is that it requires structural change and that notions of empowerment being pursued from a health reform perspective are incapable of leading to action to achieve real social change (Anderson, J. M., 1996). In Chapter 7 we reflect on the potential connection between strategies for empowerment and strategies to achieve real change in the conditions within which people experiencing severe psychological distress live their lives.

Conclusion

In this opening chapter we have identified the various dimensions of disempowerment experienced by people living with psychological distress and have outlined different ways in which the notion of empowerment might be understood. Summing up these different perspectives on empowerment we can suggest that a comprehensive view of empowerment is that it equals transformation. This transformation will need to take place in many different locations if real change in peoples' lives is to be achieved. Empowerment can be considered to comprise:

- personal growth and development;
- transformation within social groups, for example families;

- gaining greater control over life choices;
- increased influence over services received individually;
- increased influence in determining the nature of services available to all those sharing similar circumstances or characteristics;
- resistance to and subversion of dominant discourses and practices;
- gaining a presence within political systems from which you have been excluded;
- a means of achieving structural change: reducing inequalities;
- a means to health improvement;
- a process of developing and valuing different knowledges – linking knowledge and action – praxis.

We will seek to address each of these dimensions in our exploration of strategies for empowerment in the remaining chapters of this book.

2

From lunatics to survivors

The history of the mental health users movement in the UK remains sparsely documented, a function perhaps of its consciously informal nature and its relative recency. Writing in 1991 Rogers and Pilgrim (p. 130), also suggest that 'developments in Britain are not as advanced as in other countries'. They considered that this might reflect both the lack of as strong a tradition of participatory democracy as in most other developed European states and the UK's insularity towards those continental influences. It is the ambitious aim of this chapter to trace the evolution of the movement in the UK and to offer an analysis of those influences that have shaped it. This will involve brief examination of changes in the UK's political and social structure and the influence of developments elsewhere, both in Europe and further afield. The chapter continues with a review of the current nature of the movement and reflects upon the similarities and differences between the objectives and nature of the diverse groups that constitute the movement – including between those that might be distinguished as users or survivors and those characterised as carers or relatives. It concludes with a brief examination of changes within the state that have extended opportunities for the service user movement to influence those services that most impact upon service users' lives.

There have always been individuals described as 'mad' or 'mentally ill' who have been critical of the treatment meted out to them by society. It has not always been easy for them to make their voices heard. Brandon (1991) traces accounts from the seventeenth century through to the nineteenth but makes the point that 'none of the few lunatics whose writings survive were poor'. Most were aristocrats or 'wounded healers'. Extreme differences are highlighted between the nineteenth-century poet John Clare's perception of the asylum in which he spent his later years and that of its superintendent. Clare experienced this as similar to prison or slavery, while the superintendent saw Clare as enjoying perfect liberty in a rural idyll. Brandon (op. cit.) also relates Timothy Rogers' earlier view of how difficult it was to understand melancholly (*sic.*) other than by experience. Yet these accounts remained almost entirely individual writings and would only have been accessible to a few. The first sign of collective action could perhaps be seen as the formation in 1845 of the Alleged Lunatics' Friends Society by John Percival and others. Percival had previously written of his own experiences in madhouses and the group went on to figure in campaigns to reform the Victorian asylums.

It was not, of course, only lack of opportunity to put forward their views that led to the voices of asylum inmates going largely unheeded. The Victorian period saw a cementing of the revolution in ideas associated with the Enlightenment in the eighteenth century. Subsequently, in many areas of life, rational science replaced religious beliefs in offering both explanations for dysfunctions in society and the individual and a basis for possible rectification of the problem. In particular this period saw the emergence of a branch of the new medicine, called psychiatry, which shared the basic philosophical/theoretical outlook of the new science. Busfield (1986) refers to this way of thinking as the liberal-scientific conception of medicine.

The emphasis on science is important. First it implies that the origin of mental illness and the role of intervention can be studied using the methods of observation and logical inference that form the basis of natural science. As such it is based on 'fact', not value, and its definition is seen as independent of culture or social context. This has both political and organisational implications. It provides justification for the separation of medicine as a discipline and for the retention of power over defining and treating 'mental illness' outside political or popular control. Only experts trained within the closed systems of professional, clinical science and whose practice is regulated within such systems, are given the authority to make decisions – not only about the clinical care of mental patients, but also about the circumstances in which their liberty may be constrained.

The focus on physical science and its reliance on physical observation also gives rise to another important characteristic – the biological focus of medicine. While medicine is reluctant or finds it difficult to come up with a clear general definition of illness, it is based on a biological notion that the body is an organic system and illness occurs when it deviates from usual levels of functioning. In turn intervention is concerned with the physical – the internal. It is the organism not its environment that receives attention. As such there is a strong element of individualism in intervention – a focus on one to one work, on the treatment of individual patients.

The focus on biologically based intervention also militates for what we call the motor vehicle mechanic view of intervention. There is no need to view the patient as a whole person, rather the task is to find the part that is not working properly and repair or replace it. This in turn leads to a commitment to technology and the search for the 'magic bullet'. In this context, and compounded by the ideas about the impaired ability of those undergoing severe psychological distress to exercise autonomy discussed in Chapter 1, it is easy to see how there was little to be gained from listening to the views of those who did not share these expert insights.

The only real alternative to the scientific dominance of psychiatry which emerged towards the end of the Victorian period was located in the asylum reform movement. This was dominated, like others during this period, by a few dissident 'experts' and the 'great and the good'. This phil-anthropic tradition was reflected in the three major voluntary associations that became the focus of popular voice from outside the developing mental health system in the first quarter of the twentieth century:

- the Central Association for Mental Welfare (founded in 1913), which had a focus on developing volunteer-run mental health services;
- the National Council for Mental Hygiene (founded in 1922), which concentrated on educational and preventive work;
- the Child Guidance Council (founded in 1927), which promoted child guidance clinics.

These groups had different foci but could all be seen as part of the British mental hygiene movement. As such they were concerned to promote mental health and not just concerned with illness. They also recognised the role of social factors in shaping mental health problems and in determining who received treatment. However, they retained a commitment to science, which tended to exclude those who were not 'experts' from debates about the origins and appropriate response to distress. They also adopted rather moralistic positions towards those experiencing distress and placed much faith in professionals, albeit a wider range of professionals than simply clinicians (Crossley, 1998). There was little room here for a significant users' voice.

A major challenge to the scientific explanations of mental illness was provided by the emergence of 'shell shock' among a huge number of soldiers fighting in the First World War. By the end of the war, 80,000 soldiers experiencing a variety of symptoms (both physical and psycho-logical) had passed through army medical establishments. By this time there were 20 army hospitals specifically for such 'cases' (Showalter, 1987). These cases both presented a challenge to psychiatrists seeking explanations of the cause of the symptoms being experienced by these men and challenged their capacity to treat them. One 'treatment' devised to 'cure' the symptoms of shell shock was that of electric shocks, delivered directly to the throats of men who had become mute to force them to speak. The delivery of this treatment was a clear expression of the exercise of power over patients, applied in the absence of any convincing 'scientific' explanation of the cause of the problem or efficacy of the treatment (Showalter, ibid.: 176–8).

Individual descriptions of treatment in asylums continued to emerge – for example, in the poetry of Wilfred Owen, admitted himself for the treatment of shell shock, and the writing of Janet Frame. Frame's reflections on her experience in English psychiatric hospitals provide one of the earliest insights into concerns about electro-convulsive therapy (ECT). This was developed in the late 1930s in Italy and introduced to England in 1940 and was to become a major target for user and survivor movements in later years.

Nonetheless, the voices of psychiatric patients had relatively little public impact in the period between the World Wars and much of what has been learnt about their perceptions of life in asylums in the 1920s and 30s comes from retrospective accounts that emerged much later.

Psychiatry and the welfare state

The years immediately following the Second World War, when what we now consider to be the modern welfare state came into being, saw no great change. The nature of the National Health Service which emerged in this period of collective optimism was substantially determined by the powerful medical lobbies. Indeed there developed in the 1950s a considerable level of shared public and governmental confidence in welfare state professionals such as teachers, doctors and welfare workers. They were seen as the people most able to make appropriate judgements about the needs of service users and how they should be met. The senior members of the profession and their managers and administrators were in turn trusted to make the important strategic planning and management decisions that had medium and long-term consequences for the shape of the services. 'Service user' and 'public' views were best expressed through their influence on their elected representatives at local and central government level. This confidence in welfare state professionals was exemplified, in the field of mental health, by the 1959 Mental Health Act. This removed certain legal constraints on decisions about the compulsory detention and treatment of psychiatric patients and placed them firmly in the hands of doctors.

Also immediately post-war, the three major voluntary mental health organisations had merged, with Government encouragement, to become the National Association for Mental Health. Its membership continued to be predominantly middle class and educated and to include many doctors and other professionals. It focused on education via publication, demonstration projects and worker training and, given the context, it is not surprising that its targets were often professionals and politicians, with whom it carried considerable influence.

There were criticisms during this period of the paternalism inherent in the way welfare services were run (for example Wootton, 1958) and Crossley (1998: 482) refers to 'some very early indications of an emerging user voice (towards which NAMH showed some degree of receptivity)'. They stimulated little significant change, however, and even in the late 1960s something as simple as a consumer survey continued to be seen as an exciting departure.

All this altered in the 1960s and early 1970s when it is possible to see a range of related influences, from both within the UK and internationally, converging to produce significant change. This was a period of economic growth and consolidation of the welfare state. It was also a period in which the growth of and wider access to the mass media and the publication of both academic and popular accounts of the effects of welfare services led to a questioning of their efficacy. Social movements such as the women's movement and civil rights movements started to develop powerful critiques of the assumptions underpinning social policy. They also made connections between the experiences of women and black people in their private lives and the paternalist and racist ideologies driving public policy making.

Academic analyses of the nature and impact of institutional practices on the lives of those contained within them, such as Goffman's (1968) influential· work, were backed up by empirical research (Miller and Gwynne, 1972), personal accounts of those living and working in such institutions (Ryan and Thomas, 1980) and the reports of official inquiries prompted by reports of abusive and de-humanising practices (for example the Committee of Inquiry into Farleigh Hospital of 1971). These were seen as geared to the needs of the staff and the institution itself rather than those of the service user. These critiques and exposures concerned institutions for people with physical disabilities, older people and people with learning disabilities, as well as psychiatric hospitals.

The result of depersonalised practices was seen to be not only to deny those in the institution access to opportunities to exercise choice and power but to magnify their disadvantage, not least through the process some termed 'learned helplessness' (Seligman, 1975; Fennell, 1977). Another perspective emerged from the work of Wolfensberger (1972), who developed the concept of 'normalisation'. The poor quality segregated systems of support offered to groups of people identified as having 'special needs' were considered to reinforce the societal devaluation and the diminished self-perception of members of those groups. The principles of normalisation in contrast imply the development of services that challenge those perceptions and minimise stigma by giving opportunities for service users to experience the rights and responsibilities which are open to the rest of society.

There were also developments which served to undermine confidence in psychiatry and its scientific base. There were several reports on hospital scandals (for example at Ely in 1969; Farleigh in 1971 and Whittingham in 1972), which focused upon poor physical conditions, draconian restrictions on individuals, little evidence of cure or even active treatment on some wards and, in extreme cases, some evidence of physical abuse. There was also research providing evidence of more limited achievements by psychiatric interventions (certainly in terms of cure) than the optimists argued. More disturbing was evidence of significant inconsistency in diagnosis and arguably more mischievous experiments like Rosenhan's report of volunteers faking symptoms and being admitted to hospitals with psychiatric diagnoses (Rosenhan, 1973: Sheldon, 1984).

This period also saw the development of oppositional voices within the psychiatric and related professions, who argued in various ways that it was necessary to recognise that the symptoms of mental distress reflected an individual's life experiences. Hence it was appropriate to focus not on symptoms but on the meaning behind them. This could only be achieved by listening to the voice of those experiencing distress. These ideas are often described collectively as anti-psychiatry – 'a loose and woolly label to describe... pioneering ways of accepting the consumers as an intelligible human being, no matter how "mad"' (Brandon, 1991: 42). Although Brandon (and others) viewed anti-psychiatry as a pioneering breakthrough in challenging psychiatric orthodoxy, the anti-psychiatrists were themselves psychiatrists. As such, they were arguably exercising just as much power and control over their patients as more traditional practitioners. Anti-psychiatry was a professionally-led critique – the voices claiming the right to re-define the nature of the experience of schizophrenia were not those who had been assigned the diagnosis, but academics and practitioners. Thus a book entitled *The Politics of Mental Health*, published in the series *Critical Texts in Social Work and the Welfare State* was written collectively by a 'radical mental health group' comprising social workers, a day centre worker and psychologists (Banton *et al.*, 1985). While all were receiving psychoanalysis or psychoanalytic psychotherapy, this was in the tradition of therapist being required to undergo therapy, rather than an indication that they were 'users of mental health services'. This book can be contrasted with *The Politics of Disablement*, published in the same series and authored by Mike Oliver, a disabled man who was subsequently appointed to a Chair in Disability Studies at the University of Greenwich (Oliver, 1990). The radical analysis of mental health was being provided, even into the mid-1980s, primarily by radical practitioners not by those using mental health services.

The 1970s also saw an upsurge in concern for individual freedom and the civil rights of the individual. In the USA and Europe there was great pressure on governments to review restrictions on the liberty of citizens and popular movements for civil rights developed in many countries, challenging many aspects of social and political life. In Britain the National Campaign for Civil Liberties, led by Director Tony Smythe, was at the centre of many of these struggles. In 1973 he became Director of NAMH, which later called itself MIND. Their legal director was an American lawyer, Larry Gostin, who was very concerned with liberties (or restrictions upon them) within the mental health system in the UK. The name change – the change to names with more 'market impact' was fashionable at the time – also marked a change in style to one more overtly concerned with citizenship and civil rights of people experiencing severe mental distress.

This American influence is not a coincidence. The 1960s in the USA saw a major process of de-institutionalisation in psychiatry and the development of an influential consumer movement that demanded greater sensitivity to the expressed needs of consumers of the products and services offered both by private enterprises and government agencies. Often starting with small local groups, the mental health service users movement blossomed and gave rise to organisations such as the

Insane Liberation Front and the National Alliance of Mental Patients (later known as the National Alliance of Psychiatric Survivors). Their initial campaigns focused first on the unacceptability of involuntary commitment and treatment and later a wider critique of the helping process. They were particularly concerned with the iatrogenic effects of medication; the way that services fostered dependency rather than self-determination; and the focus of psychiatric discourse on symptoms and diagnosis rather than the 'real problems' experienced by service users – such as stigma, lack of employment, poverty and difficulties in relationships (Segal *et al.*, 1993).

There also developed in the USA another powerful consumer lobby – local and regional groups representing the families of those in distress – which gave rise in 1979 to the National Alliance for the Mentally Ill. Similar interests were also represented by broader-based groups like the National Mental Health Consumers Association which encompassed both those experiencing distress and their carers. These groups accepted the medical model of mental illness but nonetheless recognised the disempowering influence of professional control for both patients and relatives and championed consumer-controlled alternatives. One indication of the impact of these organisations was the blossoming of self-help organisations and the adoption of the idea of 'self-determination' as a guiding principle for the Community Support Program launched by the National Institute of Mental Health in 1977 (McLean, 1995).

Out of these influences, there gradually emerged in the UK a drive for a stronger role for the users of public services, including mental health services, in shaping the interventions that had an important impact on their lives. What was not always understood at this point was that service providers throughout the public sector often had very different motivations for and expectations of this involvement than service users themselves. Nor was it always explicitly recognised that there were important differences in the interests of the different groups who could be seen as service users.

An early example of such differences in perception came with the Skeffington initiatives in planning and the 'public involvement' this heralded. Many remember this as a series of public relations road shows and the chance to attend not always full public meetings in poorly heated school buildings where council officials talked down to the audience in defending plans that were 99 per cent certain to be implemented anyway. Well-organised groups, aided and abetted usually by sympathetic lawyers and/or academics from the planning disciplines, occasionally achieved major publicity and sometimes change. However, the role always seemed to be a reactive one, which was inevitably limited in effect.

Even where there was enthusiasm from within public services to encourage service user involvement, the motivations were not uniform. Critiques of institutionalised and professional power gave rise to concerns to extend civil liberties and participative democracy – the 'democratic imperative' – but also to ideas about empowering individuals as part of their resistance to the debilitating effects of disability or perceived mental illness – the 'therapeutic imperative'. The tensions between these sometimes complementary but different objectives have not always been recognised (Clayton, 1988). Brandon sees this confusion as a continuing issue. Talking about consultation with service users in 1986 he argued, 'the purposes of a number of meetings seemed obscure – a complex mixture of politics and therapy. This heady and confusing mixture is a major problem in mental illness services' (1991: 63).

Arguably the most important developments were not having taking place within UK mental health services – but among service users themselves who began to organise autonomously. The most well known of these early organisations were the Mental Patients Union and Community Organisation for Psychiatric Emergencies, which both formed in the early 1970s. While they gained some media attention they neither consolidated nor had the impact at this stage of similar organisations in the USA or the Netherlands (Rogers and Pilgrim, 1991).

In Holland the '*clientenbond*' was formed in 1971 following a decision to sack a respected psychiatrist from a children's psychiatric unit. Originally comprising parents who got together to resist this decision, within two years the *clientenbond* shifted to become a radical users' movement which started to demand greater say in the running of psychiatric hospitals. Patient advocacy became well established during the early 1980s. The National Foundation of Patient Advocates was established in 1981 after discussion involving organisations concerned with patients' rights, government bodies and psychiatric hospitals. Patient advocates are recruited by the Foundation and all psychiatric hospitals must allow them access to premises, patients and staff. In addition to advocates working individually with patients, the early activities of the *clientenbond* led to the establishment of patients' councils in hospitals. In 1981 the National Association of Patients Councils was created to give support and guidance to councils being established in individual hospitals. The developments in Holland had a direct impact on the emerging UK service user movement during the mid-1980s as we show below.

Proliferation and diversification

The late 1970s until the present day have seen discernible developments in the emerging picture of public and user challenge to professional and 'official' decision making. At a societal level there has been an extended period of economic stagnation and the lengthy tenure of a Conservative government, one of whose central projects was the dismantling of the welfare state. This in turn opened up opportunities for those questioning the reliance of that welfare provision on professional power. This was reflected not only by increased opportunities for users of services to influence important welfare state decisions (and indeed growing legislative sanction for such developments), but also a growth in the size and effectiveness of the autonomous service user movement.

Partly this can be ascribed to a situation of political monopoly, constructed by a strong central government, which sought to limit the impact of difference offered within local democracy, and ineffective opposition from traditional opposition parties and the trades union movement. Within this context many groups felt their interests unrepresented within the conventional political sphere and developed autonomous and innovative forms of organisation and action. As service user organisations and their interventions developed, differences in interest became apparent and a process of diversification began that offered representation to different interests within the broad concerns of service users. Greater awareness also began to develop of differences in perception of what user involvement or participation implied to different actors within health and welfare services and the political bodies that controlled them.

The UK mental health service users movement really took off in the mid-1980s and like other social movements took many organisational forms. Such variations reflect philosophical differences, differences in origin and orientation towards local or national impact. Nor can all organisations easily be classified according to these dimensions as the development of each reflects the various influences that have shaped the movement.

One of the earliest groups to develop was Nottingham Advocacy Group (NAG) which since 1986 has offered an extensive local programme of collective self-advocacy (patients' councils), citizen advocacy and individual patient (or legal) advocacy. Its origins have been traced variously to the highlighting, within Nottingham MIND and a local law centre, of the concerns of disparate groups of service users and ex-service users (Mullender, 1991), to patients' councils run by staff on hospital wards and to the influence of contact with Dutch users (Gell, 1987). NAG has not only provided an example and support for those developing similar locally based models of advocacy, including Birmingham's User Voice, but activists within NAG have shown a national orientation in directly supporting those developments in other parts of the country.

NAG is an example of an independent organisation within the service users movement that, at least in part, grew out of state sponsored activity and which continues to be sustained and given legitimacy by its relationship with state provision. Now patients' councils and user groups are becoming increasingly widespread within mental health services as service providers seek feedback from the direct users of their services. Groups have been established on hospital wards, even in the less than encouraging context of high security special hospitals, among users of day centres and in rehabilitation hostels. Service providers have also funded advocacy services run by voluntary agencies and independent user groups. For example, at Rampton Special Hospital there is a Patients' Council which receives support from an independent advocacy service provided by MACA (The Mental Aftercare Association). In addition to the project manager and administrator there are four advocacy workers, including one focusing on women's experiences within the special hospital and another who works with African-Caribbean patients. Advocacy addresses a wide range of experiences within a high secure environment that places inevitable constraints on individual autonomy while also constituting 'home' for long periods of people's lives (http://www.space.pipex.com/advocacy/). Similar developments have taken place at both Ashworth and Broadmoor, the other two high security hospitals in England.

Other user-based organisations have developed from within the traditional voluntary sector. MIND itself has changed. Its local associations remain significant providers of supported housing, crisis help-lines, drop-in centres, counselling, befriending, legal advice, advocacy and employment and training schemes. Many are supported by paid staff, significant numbers of whom describe themselves as service users or ex-service users, and emphasis is placed on facilitating involvement of the users of those services in their management.

The MIND/World Federation of Mental Health conference of 1985 was a significant event in the development of the UK users' movement as it was this event which introduced users in the UK to the Dutch developments. Three years later MIND co-sponsored a conference called 'Common Concerns' with East Sussex Social Services Department and Brighton Health Authority that brought together service users and professionals. It was an event which provoked what has been described as 'turbulent' discussion as professionals found themselves directly challenged by service users (Hepplewhite, 1988).

MIND continues to be a campaigning organisation and is committed to engaging its members, the public and professionals in the issues concerning people experiencing mental distress. Its RESPECT campaign, launched in 1998, is an educational campaign aimed at gathering support for the ending of discrimination on mental health grounds. It focuses upon discrimination against people experiencing mental distress in the public eye, in working life and as citizens. It involves positive images – early publicity, for example, focused upon Andrew Elston, a service user who stood in the general election at Hammersmith and Fulham – as well as targeting specific examples of discrimination and misinformation.

Having a direct input into policy also remains an important goal. MIND is often called upon to offer advice to Government, health and local authorities on good practice, developments in mental health care and possible legislative changes. The extent to which that represents a users' voice is open to question. MIND's membership comprises of mental health service users themselves, concerned professionals and other concerned citizens.

In order to ensure that users had a separate voice within MIND, MINDLINK was established in 1988. Within four years it had achieved a membership of over 700, claiming to be the largest user or survivor-only national network. MINDLINK itself operates at both local and national level and members have played a leading role in campaigns such as the 'Stress on Women' campaign. This sought to expose and achieve action on women's experiences within the mental health system as well as the factors affecting their experience of psychological distress. Its location within MIND was considered to limit its capacity to act as an independent campaigning organisation. However, it was seen to provide an important focus for users to participate more actively within MIND's work and to ensure that MIND itself adopted the principles of user involvement in its decision-making structures. MINDLINK has a role both in ensuring users' perspectives are influential in campaigning activities and in representing the interests of people who use services provided by MIND.

Nonetheless, some members of the service user movement still perceive MIND as an organisation dominated by its professional members. Partly this reflects a tension between different organisational goals. Influence on policy requires a certain level of professional presentation and compromise that can sit uneasily with a commitment to open discussion and participation in policy development – 'This has had the effect of releasing an antagonism between the paternalism and advocacy of the original organisation and the aspirations for autonomy and self-advocacy on the part of the user representatives that they encourage' (Rogers and Pilgrim, 1991: 143). This was seen starkly in the controversy sparked at the 1988 AGM by the election of an ex-patient to vice-chair in preference to an eminent psychiatrist. It is a tension that confronts the service user movement as a whole.

Just as in the USA, another form of 'consumer' lobby has also developed in strength in the UK – that of the families of those experiencing distress. The best known of these organisations is the National Schizophrenia Fellowship (NSF), which was formed in 1972. By the 1990s NSF had grown to rival MIND in size and influence with a network of over 160 carer and 40 user ('Voices Forum') support groups. It, too, is a service provider and supports advice and information centres, supported housing schemes, employment programmes, respite care projects, day centres and drop-in facilities. NSF is also involved in national campaigning, advice and advocacy, research, publication and training. Its web pages state that 'NSF exists to improve the lives of everyone affected by severe mental illnesses by providing quality support, services and information and by influencing local, regional and national policies' (http://www.nsf.org.uk/).

NSF does of course share some interests with MIND and the service user movement. However, the relative balance of user and carer groups gives a clue to its main concern, which is with the carers of people with mental health problems. This was particularly starkly revealed during the early 1990s debate over the proposal to extend the powers to provide compulsory treatment to include certain categories of people who were not compulsorily detained in hospital. These 'Community Treatment Orders' were supported vigorously by NSF but opposed by the Voices Forum network of user groups that it supports. NSF not surprisingly has relatively little interest in users' rights and particularly has campaigned to keep psychiatric hospitals open. This has been a central focus of their recent campaign 'What's going Wrong?' and their report '£500 Million More'. While NSF do recognise to an extent the need for better community care services, there is an inevitable unease in any alliances involving NSF and the service user movement.

Nonetheless, the organisation has employed a user of mental health services to act as a trainer, advisor and scrutineer of policy and consultation documents. In 1992 they produced a booklet on 'How to Involve Users and Carers', arguing that this would result in:

- better understanding among staff of the full effects of mental illness or their severe illness on users and their families;
- better targeted services based on identified needs;
- better working relationships between staff, users and carers;
- a greater sense of 'ownership of services' (Took, n.d).

Important though the emergence of groups of users developing from activities within service systems and from voluntary organisations may be to the user movement as a whole, many other people who identify themselves as survivors, users or consumers of mental health services have developed their own groups and organisations outside of those links. Such organisations now exist at local and national level and are increasingly connected through international networks. Nationally, the key organisations in the UK are Survivors Speak Out and the UK Advocacy Network (UKAN), although there are a growing number of other networks or organisations which reflects an emerging diversity within the user movement.

UKAN (as its name implies) aims to support the development of advocacy at both local and national levels. It was founded in 1991 following a conference held by the Nottingham Patients Council Support Group and the Nottingham Advocacy Group. Much of its activity has been in providing support and training to local advocacy groups and by 1998 there were over 220 groups affiliated to the network. In addition to aims relating to the development and support of user forums, patients' councils and local advocacy projects, UKAN aims:

To inform and educate the public and professionals about the work of the UK Advocacy Network and the member groups. To publicise this work in order to change public and private attitudes towards mental health service recipients and their organisations and to demonstrate the necessity for and the effectiveness of Patients' Councils, Advocacy Projects and User Forums.

Research and Development: To promote user led qualitative grounded research by and for users/survivors and the development of user led initiatives in service provision.

To be a national voice in promoting user issues and equal opportunities with a strong claim to be electorally representative of active working user led groups (http://www.inc.co.uk/~acorn/acorn/Ukanabout.htm).

Survivors Speak Out (SSO) is a large national organisation, composed of individuals and groups of survivors and allies, and is committed to collective self-advocacy. It formed in 1986 following the International Conference of the World Federation of Mental Health held in the UK. It is particularly committed to intervention at a national level and has been notably involved in the organisation of lobbies and demonstrations and made an immediate impact through its involvement with the television programme *We're Not Mad We're Angry*. 'The term survivors was chosen to portray a positive image of people in distress and people whose experience differs from, or who dissent from, society's norms.' (http://www.inc.co.uk/~acorn/acorn/survivor.htm). SSO has a more explicitly challenging approach to the medical model of mental illness than does UKAN. It also locates its objectives more directly in an analysis of the negative impact of professional power: 'SSO believes that many aspects of psychiatry actively take power away from and impose upon, individuals and that this is a major cause of increased distress.' Its objectives include promoting positive images of survivors and within the movement artists, poets, computer programmers and accountants are working in different ways to demonstrate the diverse wealth of talents represented within it. Their web pages include survivors' poetry and a booklet of this poetry has been published.

Local groups may or may not identify themselves with such umbrella organisations. Within these groups there are differences in terms of the priorities given to campaigning or advocacy and to the provision of alternative services. One example of a group concentrating on service delivery is McMurphy's in Sheffield. This took its name from the character in the film *One Flew Over the Cuckoo's Nest* and this was intended to demonstrate a rejection of traditional ways of providing mental health services. McMurphy's operates as a drop-in centre, primarily for younger people with mental health problems, which is run entirely by its members. One part of the centre is for women only. While members provide informal advocacy for each other on occasion, the emphasis is on providing an alternative space where members can spend time and engage in conversations and activities if they wish to, rather than seeking to influence the nature of services provided by statutory agencies. It was described in a review produced in 1995 as being:

> based on the principles of self-help and mutual support and is both developed and run by those who use it. It offers opportunities to meet friends, to socialise and to share problems if necessary. We attempt to strengthen individuals' social networks in an attempt to combat the social alienation of the loss of confidence, demoralisation, aimlessness and despair often associated with mental health problems. (McMurphy's, 1996)

Each of these different forms of organisation gives rise to different possibilities for action and to different implications for empowerment that are explored in detail in Chapter 3.

Developments within the state

Parallel to these developments within service user movements in the late 1970s and early 1980s, opportunities opened up for users to exercise their voice within the formal state apparatus. Dissatisfaction with the extent to which service users' wishes and needs were reflected within welfare provision was reflected by attempts to change the way they were planned and delivered. One example was the movement promoting 'patch social work'. This involved the allocation of workers to particular individual geographical areas so that they might get to know better the strengths and weaknesses of specific locations. Hence they would be able to provide services that made best use of existing community strengths as well as addressing their weaknesses. This led to experiments involving groups of service users and the public (the distinction was not always too clearly made) in decision-making, or at least advisory, forums. User surveys also became popular.

The three central aims of the patch movement were to: find out more about what service users wanted; open up professional activities to direct scrutiny by service users; and share power over some of the activities of social services departments. It would be wrong to go overboard about actual successes in the patch movement, particularly as regards power-sharing, but it did create a challenge to prior assumptions about the passive status of users of public services. There was, however, always a distinction between those whose aim was the opening up of services to more democratic control and those for whom increased user involvement was mainly driven by the search for more appropriate, effective services – the 'managerial imperative' (Bowl and Ross, 1994).

Such distinctions were rarely openly recognised at that time and user involvement and participation remained ill-defined concepts. One consequence of this was that just about everyone appeared to be in favour, although if a closer look was taken, everyone seemed to be talking about different ideas. This was particularly true of two contested aspects of user involvement: the competing interests of different 'users'; and the extent to which power was transferred from professionals to service users.

'Patients', 'carers' and 'the public', are distinct categories of public service users whose needs and concerns are legitimate and yet different. Those experiencing mental distress have a fundamental interest in being supported, cared for in secure, welcoming surroundings, where stress is reduced and they have the maximum chance to sort through their problems with minimum long-term erosion of their lifestyle. This fundamental interest will guide their views on services for them and people like them. Ideally those services would enhance their autonomy, help to empower them and involve social workers and hospitals in very small measure.

'Carers' are naturally also concerned with reducing the stress they themselves experience and with receiving help in coping with the 'patient' (with indeed reinforcement to, respite from, and sometimes eventually replacement of their role). They will need social workers and hospitals, and while they will not want those they care for to endure unpleasant conditions, they will be less concerned with, or even sure of, their ability to exercise autonomy. As illustrated above, the tensions between these different 'patient' and 'carer' perspectives have been demonstrated by differences between 'patient' and 'carer' based service users' organisations over support for keeping psychiatric hospitals open and also over proposals for Community Treatment and Supervision Orders. The 'public' have another set of interests, concerned possibly about the patient out of altruism and a feeling of 'There but for the grace of God...,' but principally through interest in issues of public safety.

These distinctions have not always been clearly made by those championing user involvement. Even Beresford and Croft fail to make the distinction in the survey underpinning some of their earlier writing on this area (1986). The most frequent blurring is of the interests of clients and carers and claimed high levels of user involvement often turn out to concern predominantly carers (McGrath, 1989). Taylor

(1992) was among those who recognised a clear distinction between these interests. Indeed Taylor further identified the distinct interests of potential and excluded users and the need for those to be addressed within schemes for consultation.

There has also often been a failure to make another fundamental distinction in state-sponsored initiatives for the involvement of service users – that concerning the degree of devolution or power sharing. It is a failure that is also reflected in writing about the more established psychiatric consumer movement in the USA (McLean, 1995). Perhaps the most frequent form of 'involvement' has been post-hoc consultation – where, for example, draft plans are put out for comment and possible amendment. This may be all that many public service users desire and might well enhance the quality of plans or management decisions but it involves no real shift in the balance of power. Consultation can also take place at an early stage before commitments to particular courses of action have been generated. In this way service users may influence what the agenda is to be, what management decisions are to be taken and what form a plan takes. This was the model followed by Birmingham's 'Shifting the Balance' forward plan for mental health services (Coe, 1992). Service users were represented in the discussions that led to the publication of this document, although were involved in numbers too small to guarantee an impact if opposed by a professional consensus.

Croft and Beresford (1990) identified 70 per cent of user involvement initiatives within social services at the time as 'consultation' but made no distinction concerning its timing. Indeed they were probably also including the participation of service users on strategic decision-making bodies (for example, joint care planning teams and groups drawing up community care plans) and on groups responsible for the regular management of services (departmental committees, area sub-committees and committees concerned with individual resources such as day centres or residential establishments). Because these involve service users being present when decisions are taken, these have often been seen as potentially offering service users a little more power and have been classified as 'participation' rather than consultation. Consultation can also be used to describe bodies which consist only of service users but where their direct links to policy making are limited and mediated by professional groups, who make any final decision, or where the areas over which they have discretion are strictly limited by higher placed professional bodies. Many user committees in individual establishments and patients councils in hospitals can be seen in this way.

A different strategy for involvement involves service users in 'joint working' with professional administrators and professionals. This is conceivable, for example, within the framework of a strategic planning exercise like 'Shifting the Balance' if conducted as a combined enterprise with approximately equal weighting in representation with users' organisations. Lord (1989) and Church and Reville (1989) make a similar distinction in examining the development of user involvement initiatives in Canada in stressing the differences between listening to users – what Church and Reville classify as 'user participation' – and working with them in partnerships and coalitions. A further step involves handing over power to facilitate user control – for example, in the form of transfer of a building and funds to be spent, perhaps even local authority employees on secondment to be managed.

These developments in opening up opportunities for service users to become involved in state provision within the UK have been given national government sanction through a succession of pieces of legislation. These have advocated greater user involvement in decisions about service development and allocation – with the espoused aim of ensuring that services are more responsive to the needs of service users. The White Paper on community care, *Caring for People: Community Care into the Next Decade and Beyond*, for example, was expressly concerned with giving '...people a greater individual say in how they live their lives and the services they need to help them do so' (DoH, 1989: 4).

The subsequent NHS and Community Care Act 1990 and guidance were curiously limited in their definition of the limits and nature of that participation, however, and fell some way short of conferring specific rights on service users and carers. Indeed the broad brush nature of the new legislative demands meant that social services departments and health authorities had considerable scope for their own interpretations of what facilitating user involvement meant in practice. Hence each social services department had a responsibility to establish procedures for receiving comments and complaints from service users and to ensure that consumer choice and involvement were enhanced. There was, however, no specific mandate concerning how the procedures should be set up or their substance. Health authorities were similarly exhorted by the short-lived National Health Service Management Executive to become 'Champions of the People' (NHSME, 1992). They were to involve the public generally and sub-sections of it in determining health needs as a basis on which services should be purchased and commissioned. Early responses to this indicated little more than a proliferation of surveys and some focus-group discussions.

Neither the community care White Paper nor the attendant policy guidelines had sections which looked specifically at the issue of user or carer involvement and participation or at the concepts of advocacy or self-advocacy. The implication appeared to be that, having stated at the beginning that the new-look community care was about giving more say to users and carers, the structural changes required by the legislation would, in some mysterious way, automatically produce a cultural shift within purchaser and provider agencies, to a more user-centred approach.

Nevertheless, the 1990s have seen a continuation of official commitment to involving service users and citizens within decision-making processes in health and social care services (and in public services and public policy making more generally). Encouragement to user involvement in the context of mental health has since been provided in various documents, for example *The Health of the Nation* initiative (DoH, 1992) and the mental health nursing review *Working in Partnership* (DoH, 1994). *Building Bridges* (DoH, 1995) even describes user involvement as an accepted requirement of good practice.

The complex interactions between the diverse forms of the user or survivor movement and these changes within the state, and their implications for empowerment strategies, are the theme of Chapter 3.

3

Strategies for empowerment

As we discussed in Chapter 2, self-organisation among people who use mental health services or who have been designated as 'mad' or 'mentally ill' is not an entirely new phenomenon. Nevertheless, the development of both autonomous action on the part of mental health service users, and action from within service systems to in some way 'involve' service users has gathered pace since the 1980s. These two different movements: one based in experiences of oppression, of being unheard and of having civil rights violated, the other deriving from consumerist notions of 'listening to the customer' are paralleled in the context of other areas of public policy and service delivery in the UK and elsewhere (see for example Gyford, 1991; McLean, 1995; Trainor *et al.*, 1997; Barnes *et al.*, 1998, 1999a and b). As the mental health user movement has developed in the context of, first, neo-liberal notions of the benefits of welfare markets, and with the advent of a 'New Labour' government in the UK in 1997, an emerging discourse of 'partnership' between the makers and subjects of public policy, different models of organising and different priorities for action have emerged within the movement.

In this chapter we discuss key differences in the objectives and strategies within the mental health user movement at the end of the twentieth century. Our emphasis is on the UK, but we also draw on experience elsewhere which suggests that differences in the nature of the system of welfare within societies may influence the possibilities open to user movements and the decisions they make about objectives and strategies. We start with a consideration of the different sites within which action is being taken among mental health service users. This illustrate something of the diversity of the contemporary movement.

Sites of action among mental health service users in the UK: implications and dilemmas

We can identify at least five different locations within which action is being pursued among mental health service users. These different locations have implications for the change strategies being pursued and for their impact.

Voluntary action: the distinction between 'for' and 'of'

Within the disabled people's movement the distinction between organisations of and for disabled people is a crucial way of distinguishing 'traditional' voluntary action and action controlled by disabled people. The emergence of the disabled people's movement was as much a response to the paternalism of 'do gooding' voluntary organisations as it was to the exclusionary policies of the state welfare sector. The challenge offered by the 'of' movement subsequently caused some traditional organisations 'for' disabled people to reflect on their own constitutions and objectives, and to establish their own 'user forums' as part of their decision making structures. The Leonard Cheshire Foundation which is a major service provider for disabled people is one such organisation.

Within the mental health field some voluntary organisations whose membership has reflected the range of interests within the mental health system also saw the need to develop user focused or user led groups and activities under their umbrella. Thus MINDLINK developed under the umbrella of MIND with both national and regional organisations reflecting the organisation of MIND as a whole. Even the National Schizophrenia Fellowship, an organisation funded primarily to reflect the interests of the families of people with a diagnosis of schizophrenia, supported the development of the 'Voices' network which brought together 'sufferers' themselves. While MINDLINK and Voices might be considered organisations *of* mental health service users, their location within organisations *for* does affect their capacity to reflect unequivocally the views and experiences of users.

In particular the approach advocated by the NSF Voices groups is that of joint working between mental health workers, users and carers. While the right of users *not* to have their carers involved in agreeing individual care plans is recognised (Took, n.d), the starting point for NSF is that carers are key stakeholders in decision making and that their interests should be powerfully represented within decision making about mental health services.

As well as evidence that national voluntary organisations are seeking to respond to principles of user involvement, there are an increasing number of voluntary organisations at a local level which are seeking to base their activities in collective and democratic principles. It is sometimes difficult to draw a firm line between 'voluntary' organisations and action within the sphere of civil society based in community action and community development principles. For example, Forty Second Street in Manchester works with young people who experience mental health problems. It has its roots in participatory models of youth work and aims to enable young people to strengthen their collective voice not only within but beyond the organisation (Batsleer, 1999).

User-focused action within voluntary organisations that are not under the direct control of users probably has more of the characteristics of user involvement which has developed in the context of statutory service commissioning and providing, than of the autonomous action of organisations 'of' disabled people which is based on the principle that direct control is a prerequisite for emancipation. However, the re-emergence of community development as a practice in both local government and the health service, as well as the voluntary sector, suggests there may be a blurring of boundaries between different models of participation being pursued in different contexts. We will return to this in the final chapter.

Separate organisation

People who identify themselves as survivors, users or consumers of mental health services have developed their own groups and organisations separate from service systems and from voluntary organisations *for* rather than *of*. Such organisations now exist at local and national level and are increasingly linked in international networks. As we have seen, nationally, the key organisations in the UK are Survivors Speak Out and the UK Advocacy Network (UKAN), although there are a growing number of other networks or organisations which reflect an emerging diversity within the user movement. For example, the Hearing Voices network has provided a forum within which people who hear voices can develop alternative understandings and ways of responding to and dealing with these experiences from those offered by the medical profession. Other groups have developed based around the experience of eating disorders, or among people who express their distress through self-harm.

The objectives of such groups include personal empowerment through valuing the experience and knowledge of survivors as well as by strengthening social networks and demonstrating the possibilities of collective action. They seek empowerment within the mental health system by challenging professional control and demonstrating alternative models of support for people experiencing distress. They aim to achieve a presence at national level in order to exert more political influence on mental health policy makers, and they target the domain of civil society through action intended to challenge the stigmatisation of people experiencing distress in media representations as well as in social interactions in everyday life.

They adopt a wide range of strategies in order to achieve these aims. In a study of three mental health user groups and three disabled people's groups, Barnes *et al.* (1996) identified six categories of action/strategy from an analysis of interviews with user activists:

1. *Joint working.* User groups worked with officials within individual services, at service planning level with individual health and local authorities, and some had taken part in national policy making and planning forums.

2. *Research and training.* Two of the three mental health user groups were involved in research and training initiatives intended to change the way in which professionals think about mental distress.

3. *Delivering alternatives.* One of the groups saw itself primarily in terms of providing alternative services, although all provided information and advice services and one had purchased a caravan in order to be able to offer inexpensive holidays to members.

4. *Using the market.* The separation of purchasing from provision of services was seen to offer some opportunities to influence mainstream mental health services. One way in which groups were seeking to impact upon the nature and quality of services was through influencing the content of service contracts. Groups used their contacts with people on the receiving end of services in order to monitor 'contract compliance' and to call to account providers who were not delivering what they said they would.

5. *Campaigning and politics.* One of the three mental health groups saw itself primarily as a campaigning group. Campaigning involved using media and political contacts to achieve influence, as well as the collection of evidence to support their case in dialogue with officials. One of the mental health groups had a media adviser and regularly made use of the local press to pursue its campaigns. Another group made use of local media in publicising its regular Mental Health Awareness Week.

6. *Direct action.* Direct action is a tactic used by the radical end of the user movement – in particular among disabled people. There was only one example quoted among the mental health user groups in the study when there was a spontaneous 'taking over' of a meeting discussing plans for the re-organisation of mental health services.

The expression of voice was fundamental to all the strategies being pursued by virtually all groups. Voice could be expressed through collective representation in official forums; through individual advocacy, or through campaigning, lobbying or direct action. The user group which prioritised the provision of a user-run drop-in service provided opportunities for the expression of voice through arts and poetry. Thus voice could be expressed within the system and outside it, on different occasions by the same group. The voice to be heard was variously a consumer voice; the 'expert' voice; the voice that had never been listened to; a voice calling officials to account. The groups aimed to encourage and support people to find their voices, and to ensure they were listened to.

Also underpinning all these strategies for achieving influence in different spheres was the importance of collective organisation per se as a means of enabling personal support and development to those taking part in the groups, as a source of increased legitimacy through expressing collective views, and as a forum in which experiential knowledge could be articulated and valued.

Research and education

An increasingly important aspect of separate organisation on the part of mental health service users is the way in which this is leading to the development of alternative explanations and understandings of severe psychological distress. The Hearing Voices movement is one example of this (Romme and Escher, 1993). The origin of this is in the disjuncture between people's experiences of distress and the explanations and responses they receive from psychiatric professionals. The strategy focuses not on securing immediate and specific change in particular services, but in accessing the experiential knowledge of people experiencing psychological distress in order to develop alternative models of explaining, understanding and hence responding to such experiences. While some groups have used this in the context of self-help initiatives, others have sought wider impact through user-led research disseminated within mainstream systems, or in contributing directly to the education and training of mental health professionals.

UK organisations such as the Mental Health Foundation and the Sainsbury Centre for Mental Health have employed users as researchers and policy analysts and have developed models of research which engage users as active researchers rather than place them as passive subjects of research. The 'Strategies for Living' programme supported by the Mental Health Foundation was launched with a user-led survey of alternative and complementary treatments and therapies which resulted in the publication of *Knowing our Own Minds* (Faulkner, 1997). The programme builds on the findings of that survey with the aim of exploring the diverse ways in which people live and cope with mental health problems. It also seeks to ensure that knowledge is shared and available not only to users or survivors, but also to service providers and purchasers to influence their strategy for mental health service development (http://www.mentalhealth.org.uk/s41prout.htm).

Academic institutions are increasingly involving users as educators in qualifying and post-qualifying professional courses. For example, the postgraduate Community Mental Health Programme at Birmingham University includes users both as teachers and as members of the advisory group for that programme, while the Approved Social Worker training programme run from the same university also employs service users as core trainers.

Users have also set up their own independent training and consultancy bodies. A project within a local MIND group in Solihull, West Midlands, led by an experienced user trainer developed a model of working suited both to direct empowerment objectives for the users involved, as well as the achievement of longer term objectives regarding change in the attitudes and behaviour of mental health professionals and others. Users are recruited to join a group which both receives training and works together to develop training materials. As users gain sufficient confidence they take on active roles as trainers. As well as the 'core group' there is a wider 'feeder group' of users who meet less frequently to provide an additional source of expertise to contribute to training materials development, and a wider resource in cases where people are unwell and temporarily unable to make an input.

The recognition that knowledge production is socially situated and can result in competing or contested knowledges is a central theme within contemporary social theory and social research (see for example Harding, 1991; Seidman, 1998). We discuss the place of mental health user movements in the context of these broader shifts in assumptions about the nature of knowledge and expertise in Chapter 7.

Action on mental health in other contexts

Not all those who seek change within the mental health system or in the lives of those living with severe psychological distress identify themselves primarily as users or survivors of mental health services. Groups that are based in other cultural or ethnic identities are also engaged in action concerned with mental health and empowerment (see Chapter 4). Thus, for example, in Sheffield, the Somali community became engaged in MIND's Stress on Women campaign, seeking to develop support groups for Somali women experiencing emotional distress. Similarly, the Chinese Mental Health Association (Wong and Ku, 1996) was formed to address the problems experienced among those developing mental health problems within the Chinese community. Lesbians who have experienced severe psychological distress have found support from within lesbian communities. There have been some positive examples of voluntary sector services which have sought to adopt empowering ways of working with lesbians experiencing distress (Good Practices in Mental Health, 1994).

A rather different example of action with empowerment objectives which links the experience of severe psychological distress to other aspects of socio-cultural experience is Ecoworks. Ecoworks originally developed under the umbrella of NAG in Nottingham, but developed a separate identity as an organisation concerned with addressing the underlying causes of mental distress and focusing on action outside the mainstream service system to create the conditions for mental wellbeing. It is based on an alliance between people involved in the mental health user movement and green professionals (Davey, 1999).

User involvement

All the initiatives we have considered up to now have their origins outside the sphere of the state, although their objectives include making an impact both on the nature of state services and the processes by which they are governed. But, as we discussed in Chapter 2, changes within the governance of public services have also had an important impact on opportunities for service users to become involved in decision making and have been claimed to offer openings for 'user empowerment'. In some instances a distinction between state inspired or supported action and separate organisation becomes hard to unravel as user groups configure themselves in order to engage in dialogue with commissioners and providers of mental health services. Separately organised groups sometimes receive funding from statutory organisations (local authorities and health service organisations) in the form of one-off grants or through contractual agreements to provide advocacy services. They can experience constraints on their capacity to resist or oppose the officials on whom they depend for their resources. As user groups enter into close relationships with service organisations which offer the opportunity to exercise influence from within the system, they can find themselves being expected to behave in the same way as statutory bodies. For example, in a study of mental health user groups we heard of an attempt on the part of officials to enforce 'discipline' on a group operating under the umbrella of a city-wide user council. The group was unhappy about policy in one area of the city and was campaigning against this, including writing letters to the local MP. At the same time the city-wide user representatives were engaged in dialogue with the local mental health trust about overall policy. City-wide user representatives had to point out that they did not operate the hierarchical structure of a bureaucratic organisation and that the philosophy of user–self-organisation was based in a 'bottom-up' approach to defining issues and the position to be adopted on such issues (Barnes *et al.*, 1999a).

Allies or oppressors?

A detailed discussion of an attempt to build dialogue between users and staff in an acute mental health service in Australia (Wadsworth and Epstein, 1998) explores some of the deep-seated reasons why it might be difficult for users to become empowered through working with staff within mental health services. The study revealed ways in which people who aspire to respond with compassion can end up erecting emotional defences which then get built into organisational roles and routines to control rather than enable. Thus even though staff in this project were willing to engage in dialogue with users about their experiences, much of the dialogue was dominated by expressions of staff's feelings about their work and their frustrations. The energy and resources necessary to achieving changes in attitudes and practices of staff divert attention from investment in developing skills and confidence necessary for users to empower themselves.

Groups within the mental health user movement have held, and continue to hold different views about whether they should work with allies among mental health professionals or remain separate from them. Rogers and Pilgrim (1991) highlight this as one of the key distinctions to be made between groups such as the Campaign Against Psychiatric Oppression (CAPO) which described itself as an 'abolitionist group'; SSO, which adopted a rather more ambivalent approach to working with professional allies; and Voices, which adopts a rather uncritical approach to the medical profession. More recently there have been examples of user groups forming to protect services in which both users and professionals can be considered to have a vested interest. For example 'The Friends of St Anne's Orchard' was established in response to proposals by a mental health trust's plans to move a day hospital from the building in which it was being provided to another site (http://www.st-anne's.co.uk).

The relationship between user activists and workers sympathetic to users' concerns has been a continuing theme within the mental health user movement. Both users and workers have adopted contrasting positions. At one of the early conferences in the UK which brought together user activists and mental health workers, Alec Jenner (1988) asked users to recognise what science has to offer those experiencing mental distress, as well as encouraging psychiatrists to take responsibility for supporting the user movement and learn from the insights it could offer. In contrast, user challenges to professional power and credibility have been dismissed by some psychiatrists as 'the ravings of mad men' (Barnes and Wistow, 1994b). Some groups prefer to use their energies to provide direct support to their members, or to develop alternative ways of understanding and responding to psychological distress. Others have been prepared to work with sympathetic professionals or, indeed, become involved in decision-making structures with professionals and managers who are not regarded as sympathetic, but whom the users are seeking to influence (Barnes *et al.*, 1996).

Edna Conlan, one of the founders of UKAN, addressed this tension within the UK user movement. In a paper to the World Federation for

Mental Health conference in Dublin in 1995, she described the way in which users became involved in the national Mental Health Task Force. She talked of a 'robust exchange of views' between user representatives from UKAN, Survivors Speak Out and MINDLINK, and Virginia Bottomley, then Secretary of State for Health, which had led to the invitation to meet with the head of the Task Force. Out of this developed the Task Force User Group which devised a programme of work reflecting their interests which would also meet wider Task Force objectives. She went on to reflect on the importance of taking chances in order to get into a position in which users could have the opportunity to control a high profile development programme.

Elsewhere in Europe, users have sought to develop different forums within which dialogue can take place between users, professionals and, sometimes, family members in order to build new understandings. Van der Male (1996) has described 'psychosis seminars' in Germany which have this objective, and plenary meetings in Holland which provide an open forum in which users, family members and professionals discuss local topics to initiate a process of change. A seminar in Bergen brought together Ministry of Health officials, psychiatrists, users and sympathetic academics from throughout Norway. This called for separate spaces and times in which users could be together to express their own anger and talk among themselves, but also for users to be directly involved in official bodies with responsibilities for overseeing mental health services, and for forums in which learning could take place together (Thesen, 1997). However, Jensen and Froestad (1988) have highlighted the conflicts between user organisations operating at a national level in Norway over whether collaborative or conflictual stances should be adopted in relationships with officials.

The preparedness to work with policy makers and professionals at both national and local level has continued to represent an important aspect of the movement within the UK. Indeed it would be possible to argue that major national policy development can no longer be pursued without some consultation or involvement of service users. However, it is also clear where the power continues to lie. User representatives on a national group convened by the Department of Health in 1998 to develop a national service framework for mental health services resigned when it became clear that policy developments were also going to include changes to mental health legislation based on the principle that non-compliance with medication in the community was not an option. Users (and many professionals) were very unhappy about an extension of compulsion into community settings, but, at the time of writing, it appears likely that there will be such a development and that representations from the user movement both within and outside formal consultation processes will have been insufficient to halt this.

One general point emerging from this analysis of the increasing diversity within the user/survivor movement is that this is influenced by and responsive to changes in the system itself. The health and social care system in the UK has been subject to substantial structural change during the 1980s and 1990s and there is little sign that we are entering a period of stability. The late 1990s saw a shift from the competitive ethos of markets to an appeal to partnership which has the potential to lead to horizontal change in the structuring of welfare institutions (Barnes and Prior, 2000). In the next section we discuss how changes in the policy context have affected opportunities for user involvement and empowerment. We pick up on some of the more recent changes and their likely future implications in our final chapter.

The policy context

This analysis of the different sites within which users/survivors are acting, the varied strategies adopted by the contemporary mental health user movement and the different positions taken with respect to working within or outside the system, illustrates the richness and diversity of the contemporary movement. It also suggests it is important to understand how policy and ideological contexts affect both the opportunities and constraints affecting the empowerment strategies that people experiencing psychological distress have adopted. In this section we explore in more detail aspects of the policy and service context within which the UK users/survivors movement has been developing in order to understand some of the factors which have influenced the pattern of objectives and action that has been pursued. We also provide some illustrations of differences in strategies and priorities being pursued by user movements elsewhere.

We need first of all to locate this in the context of changes in the organisation and management of health and social care heralded by the implementation of the 1990 NHS and Community Care Act. This Act not only marked official acceptance of the policy of community care (that is, that for the most part, people with mental health problems as well as physically or learning disabled people should receive support and therapeutic services in 'ordinary environments' rather than in hospitals or long-stay residential institutions), but also sought to achieve a shift away from producer interests towards the development of what was variously called a needs or user-led system of health and social care. This was to be achieved in a variety of ways, including encouraging user and carer involvement in the process of assessment by which services are accessed; requiring social services authorities to consult with users, carers and voluntary organisations during the production of community care plans; and the introduction of a complaints procedure containing an element of independent review (Barnes, 1997).

The changes introduced by the 1990 Act were part of much more widespread shifts in organisation and practice within public services introduced by the Tory governments of Margaret Thatcher and John Major. One aspect of this was an increasing emphasis on individual responsibility and individual choice rather than on the responsibility of the state to ensure the wellbeing of its citizens. Family care was seen to be the preferred option for the provision of care to 'needy' individuals. If family care was unavailable or insufficient, then people should have the option to choose to purchase care from a private supplier, or to receive support from voluntary agencies, rather than automatically assume that services would be provided directly by the state. The identification of 'carers' as an important resource in the provision of community care, as well as a recognition of the impact on family members and others of providing such support, led to the mobilisation of the carers' lobby and ultimately the passage of the 1996 Carers' Recognition and Services Act. In local government, the health service and other parts of the public sector, there were attempts to curb the powers of professionals. The mechanisms to achieve this were an increase in the powers of managers, the organisational separation of service purchasing or commissioning from direct service provision, and the recasting of public service users as customers or consumers (for example Pollitt, 1990; Flynn, 1993).

The implementation of the 1990 Act led to an increase in the number and types of initiatives to listen to the voices of service users which had been developing in more innovative authorities during the 1980s (Barnes and Wistow, 1994a). By the early 1990s user involvement was a statutory requirement which many authorities were struggling to meet (Bowl, 1996b). A variety of methods by which users might be consulted or involved in decision making at different levels started to emerge. Much of this work centred around consultation over community care plans and the related activities of service monitoring and evaluation. Glendinning and Bewley (1992) in an early study of the new community care planning process, found that much of this activity consisted of consultation with voluntary organisations, rather than the direct and active involvement of service users in the planning process. This was confirmed by other studies (for example Hoyes *et al.*, 1993), and in a summary of research into user involvement in community care Lindow and Morris (1995) identified a range of barriers to effective involvement in planning processes as well as some examples of good practice that were starting to emerge.

In addition to consultation with users and carers during the production of community care plans, an increasing emphasis on service monitoring and evaluation in both health and social care was resulting in users' views being sought through satisfaction surveys, focus groups and more interactive methods of obtaining feedback from users (for example Wilson, 1995). And as well as an increase in activity intended to explore users' views about services, the mid-1990s saw the start of more active efforts to develop user-defined outcome measures through which the impact of services could be assessed (Nocon and Qureshi, 1996).

The other main arena within which user involvement was being pursued from within service agencies was in the process of needs assessment. Once again, the research evidence demonstrates that putting into practice a process in which users felt themselves to be active participants proved difficult for workers unused to working in partnership – not least because workers undertaking needs assessment felt they were also in the position of managing demand (Ellis, 1993). The use of advocates or brokers was one way of trying to equalise the balance of power in the process of needs assessment, while another approach was to devise self-assessment tools which enabled users to go through their own needs assessment process before negotiating this with professionals (The Avon Mental Health Measure, n.d.).

Developments intended to open health service decision making processes to users lagged behind those within the social care system. But throughout the 1990s such initiatives gathered pace and examples of 'top-down' initiatives to consult with users over service planning, and to develop a practice of shared decision making in decisions about health care, are now official policy within the NHS (see for example Barnes, 1997b).

The consumerist developments of the 1980s and early 1990s cannot be equated unequivocally with a commitment to the empowerment of service users. Consumer empowerment was seen by the architects of the welfare market as one of a variety of mechanisms which could limit the power of welfare professionals. But this was in the context of a belief that state welfare itself should be 'rolled back', rather than that users should become powerful within a powerful welfare state. Managers were seen to be more likely to reflect consumer interests than were health and social care professionals and this was one of the justifications advanced for increasing the power of managers in comparison to that of direct service deliverers. Newman and Clarke (1994) relate this to the presumed ideological neutrality of management:

> Management has been identified as a transformational force counterposed to each of the old modes of power. By contrast with the professional, the manager is driven by the search for efficiency rather than abstract 'professional standards'. Compared to the bureaucrat, the manager is flexible and outward-looking. Unlike the politician, the manager inhabits the 'real world' of 'good business practices' not the realms of doctrinaire ideology. In each of these areas, the manager is also more 'customer centred' than concerned with the maintenance and development of organisational empires. (ibid.: 23)

While the philosophies underpinning consumerist initiatives from within the health and social care system may not have been consistent with the more emancipatory objectives of some sections of the users/survirvors movement, space was created within which legitimacy was granted to 'user involvement' and user groups could build relationships with service purchasers and providers through which they could hope to exert influence from within the mental health system (Gaster *et al.*, 1993; Barnes *et al.*, 1999a and b).

Many of these initiatives to listen to user voices were led by officials occupying management positions within health and social care agencies rather than by clinicians. However, we would agree with Newman and Clarke that it would be wrong to ascribe this solely to a disinterested commitment to the rights of the consumer in comparison to professional adherence to peer determined standards of practice. Mental health service users offer less of a threat to managers than they potentially do to mental health professionals. Indeed managers have sometimes acted as 'go-betweens', seeking to translate the angry responses of users into terms which may be perceived as less threatening by the doctors to whom the words are addressed. Barnes and Wistow (1994b) quote a health service manager describing how he had tried to assist in the process of expressing users' views by casting them in a language which he considered would be more likely to achieve a positive response. The user councils' worker rejected his attempts:

> I identified these issues originally in my own language and in a way that I calculated we'd get a response. Part of the problem I suspect was the language

which was seen as too soft. It was 'there appears to be an issue about this, would it be possible to?' It was that kind of stuff rather than 'this is totally not on, you are repressing us' which is determinedly expressed in the raw minutes. And so he (user council worker) didn't use it basically. He didn't use the paper, nor did he do a similar exercise for his own and so that way of identifying issues never really got off the ground. (ibid.: 532)

A distinction between the responses of managers and professionals may be more evident within the health service than within social services. There is a clearer claim to the status of 'professional' among doctors than there is to such a status on the part of social workers or other workers in the social care arena. There is also a much greater distinction between the identities of professionals and managers within the health service. A social service manager is more likely to have previously been a practising social worker than a health service manager is to have been a practising clinician. The issues typically raised with health service managers do not threaten the basis of managerial authority in the way that challenges to clinicians can do. If users complain about the food, the physical environment on wards or the range of activities available within day centres, this does not present the same degree of challenge as does a questioning of the allocation of a psychiatric diagnosis and the determination of appropriate clinical treatment. The right to make a diagnosis and prescribe a form of treatment is a core element of the professional power of doctors, jealously guarded from encroachment by other clinical staff such as nurses. Medical ethics appeal to the principle of beneficence and thus accusations by users that they are being harmed by medical interventions go right to the heart of both the values and power base of doctors. To this extent it could be hypothesised that managers might be more likely to respond sympathetically to user feedback than would doctors. But is this because they are uninterested in developing organisational empires?

Results from one in-depth study of user self-organisation and of official responses to this indicate something of the nature of the relationships which started to develop between officials and user groups (Barnes *et al.*, 1999a). At one level, local NHS and social services officials were very positive about the existence, activity and formal legitimacy accorded to user groups. They did not offer any principled objection to such groups having some place within the mental health system, recognising that a changing political and social climate required them to listen to users. They acknowledged that paternalism was no longer appropriate and they recognised that users had a type of knowledge and expertise not always possessed by either professionals or service managers. Officials saw user groups as one of a number of stakeholders whose views needed to be sought in developing and implementing policy. In such a pluralistic system, however, officials within statutory agencies reserved the right to act as 'umpire' between what they described as competing interest groups and this could (and did) result in manipulation of the particular legitimacy which might attach to user views:

> The card that you have to play all the time is user need, user preference and user view on something, and whether I am negotiating with other people inside this building, arguing with the Trust, negotiating with the Social Services Department, arguing about how we ought to spend joint finance... you in effect play the user card. (quoted in Barnes *et al.*, 1999a)

This response suggests that, far from being unconcerned about developing and maintaining organisational empires, mental health managers may see alliances with users as a route to increasing their power comparative to other players within the system. Such alliances may be cynically pursued to those ends.

Policy developments within the NHS, social services and throughout the public sector have continued to reinforce official commitment to include the perspective of service recipients in decision making. It seems unlikely that there will be a reversal of the trend towards service users becoming more active participants in individual and collective decision making about services (Barnes, 1999b). Involving 'patients, users and carers' comprises an important plank in the project to 'modernise' mental health services (DoH, 1998). The argument for this is based on research evidence of the beneficial impact of direct involvement in the process of treatment and care, the need to ensure fair treatment, to preserve autonomy and enable choice. *Modernising Mental Health Services* also makes reference to a concept which has entered official discourse as the preferred method of developing and implementing public policy: 'partnership'.

Partnership has been advocated as the mechanism for addressing a diverse range of policy problems which are themselves seen as interconnected and requiring addressing in a 'cross-cutting' manner. Partnerships between players such as local authorities, the NHS, voluntary agencies, community organisations, the private sector, the police, probation service, Training and Enterprise Councils (TECs) and others are being urged and in some cases required to address issues of health inequalities, crime and disorder, and improving educational performance. Many central government initiatives which aim to develop innovative ways of responding to social exclusion require statutory bodies to include communities as partners in this process. Health Action Zones (HAZs), for example, are encouraged to do so and some HAZs have given particular priority to community involvement as a means of achieving health improvement. However, early evidence from a national evaluation of HAZs revealed that many were very unclear about how to achieve this (Judge *et al.*, 1999).

In view of the priority being given to partnership across a range of policy areas, it is notable that, while the term partnership appears in *Modernising Mental Health Services* the concept being expressed is a narrow one. Indeed, service users themselves are not seen as partners. Rather: 'Decisions about care and treatment should be a joint endeavour between staff, patients, service users, and discussed with carers as well. Carers are partners alongside health and social services in providing care and support to people with mental health problems' (para. 4.50). This relegation of users to recipients of care from both carers and service providers makes no pretence of a commitment to empowering practice. While the voluntary and charitable sectors are recognised as valuable contributors to the network of service provision, there is no reference to user groups either as partners in determining policy and service priorities, nor as partners in delivering services. In fact the document as a whole can be read as highly conservative, not only in its approach to the nature of services required to provide 'safe, sound and supportive' mental health care, but also in its depiction of people experiencing psychological distress as recipients of care, who may be both vulnerable and a source of risk for others.

The attempt to introduce a market in health care provision within the UK demonstrated the depth of resistance to the notion that health care should be delivered by private sector agencies and that fee payment or personal insurance should be the means of financing such services. Such resistance was less marked in relation to the provision of social care services, but large-scale privatisation has been restricted to certain types of social care (such as residential care for older people). In this context there has been little evidence within the UK mental health user movement of a wholesale rejection of publicly funded and provided mental health services. The dominant objective is that of reform rather than abolition. The appeal to change has increasingly been based on the rights or fair treatment of citizens who have been excluded not only as a result of the intrinsic impact of their distress, but by public attitudes, and by the result of poor quality care (or worse) within the mental health system.

Unlike some sections of the disability movement which have concluded that the most effective way of gaining control over support services is to enter into a financial exchange relationship with those directly providing the service, mental health service users have not been arguing for direct payments to enable them to purchase their own personal support services. Nor have they been arguing to be able to exercise choice within a private market of service providers. Such choices are largely illusory for the majority of people experiencing severe psychological distress whose experience of distress is compounded by the poverty associated with unemployment. Rather they are seeking a wider range of alternative types of treatment and sources of support to be available from within the public system of health and local authority services.

The NHS and Community Care Act sought not only an expansion in the for-profit but also the not-for-profit independent sector. The response of voluntary organisations to this was ambivalent. On the one hand this appeared to provide official recognition of the significance of the role played by voluntary organisations. But for many the shift from grant giving approaches to funding to the requirement to enter into contracts or service level agreements with local authorities and health authorities was seen as fundamentally compromising their capacity to offer alternative approaches to mainstream statutory provision (Rogers, 1999). Similarly, user organisations have been reluctant to enter into contracts to provide services not only because the nature of the service is defined in terms which may be unacceptable to them, but also because the organisational implications of taking on significant service delivery responsibilities would divert them from their main purposes as advocates and could place unacceptable burdens on volunteer activists. This reluctance has been less evident in some places in North America.

Diverse objectives and strategies

In the USA and Canada a distinction has been drawn between 'consumer' organisations and 'survivor or ex-patients' organisations (for example McLean, 1995; Trainor *et al.*, 1997). This distinction is based in acceptance, or otherwise, of the medical model of mental illness. Consumer organisations are described as those which largely accept the medical classification of mental illness and hence the priority given to medical services to treat (and possibly cure) such illnesses. Thus they seek improvements in the mental health services available, but do not provide a radical critique of the model itself. Survivors' or ex-patients' groups reject the medical model and professional control over the definition and treatment of the problems experienced by those with severe emotional distress. They see user-controlled alternatives to professionally provided services as essential to achieving services which are not dominated by the medical model (for example Chamberlin, 1988).

In addition to this distinction, the North American literature identifies a strong 'self-help' movement among service users. The origins of the contemporary movement are traced to the 1930s when 'Recovery Incorporated' was established, joined in the 1950s by 'Grow' (Segal *et al.*, 1993; Trainor *et al.*, 1997). Defined by Segal *et al.* (ibid.: 705) as 'an attempt by people with a mutual problem to take control over the circumstances of their lives', self-help has a long history within the UK in the context of action among people living in poverty and oppression. But it has often been regarded as politically conservative, focusing on those subject to oppression taking action among themselves to mitigate the effects of inequality, rather than seeking social change which reduces their oppression.

The North American self-help tradition can be seen alongside the emphasis on user-controlled services as an alternative to mainstream mental health services. While there are user-controlled alternatives in the UK (such as McMurphy's) there has been some reluctance within the UK movement to move into service provision. Voluntary organisations such as MIND which have developed user groups and remain service providers recognise the dilemma associated with both providing services and being user advocates. When the response to NAG's campaign to achieve 24-hour access to crisis services was to suggest the group should itself take on the responsibility for running such services there was considerable uncertainty that this should be the way forward. User activists recognised not only the organisational implications of becoming a service providing organisation, but also the potential impact on their capacity to prioritise campaigning and advocacy. These demands and challenges are equally evident in the experience of user organisations in the USA and Canada, but in the absence of a national health service equivalent to that of the UK, there is a more highly developed tradition of raising funds and seeking planning approval for alternative service provision.

However, as McLean (1995) has shown in her in-depth study of a user-run community resource centre in the USA (discussed in more detail in Chapter 5), it is not necessarily the case that a user-run service can automatically be equated with a resource capable of contributing to the empowerment of those who use it. McLean's research suggests that the concerns of UK users that the achievement of empowerment objectives may be compromised by taking on service provision responsibilities has some justification. She suggests that the rapid growth of user-controlled services has led to an amnesia about the original emancipatory mission of the survivor movement and that such services are in danger of simply reproducing oppressive provider/consumer relationships.

In other welfare state systems there is little evidence of empowerment strategies prioritising the development of user-controlled alternatives to statutory services. For example in Norway there is felt to be a high level of commitment to a well-developed welfare state which deters service users from organising to challenge health service provision. Thus, while there is a developing mental health service users/survivors movement, there is little evidence of direct user advocacy operating within psychiatric hospitals, and it has been suggested that professionals would not accept users acting as advocates (personal communication from users in Hieronymous and We Shall Overcome in Bergen). At local level, user-led self-help and support groups such as Angstringen are developing what is called the 'new voluntary work', based in notions of mutual benefit rather than the principle of donor and recipient (Angstringen-Oslo, 1995). Hieronymous in Bergen is developing a more political analysis of the experience of service users, but has no recognised role within service planning or decision-making systems.

Trainor *et al.*'s (1997) analysis of the 'service paradigm' is useful for distinguishing action within user movements which can contribute to broad empowerment objectives, and objectives defined in the context of service provision – whether that be services provided by users themselves or by mental health professionals. Trainor and his colleagues describe the activities that resulted from a funding programme in Ontario called the Consumer/Survivor Development Initiatives (CSDI). While initial programme grants went to both fully independent consumer/survivor organisations and to mental health agency sponsored projects, criteria for accessing funds were later restricted to consumer/survivor controlled organisations. A further restriction on funding criteria was that it was not available for the provision of direct services: 'This restriction stemmed from the mandate of the Ontario initiative. The goals of the funding were twofold; they were intended to respond to calls by consumers/survivors for both a base of organisations that they controlled, and for the chance to deal in a new way with the mental health issues that they faced.' Thus an important intention of this programme was that it should be capable of stimulating alternative approaches to understanding and responding to psychological distress, rather than simply transferring responsibility for service provision to users.

Some success in this is demonstrated by the fact that, of the 36 groups funded through this programme: 93 per cent were engaged in mutual support; 83 per cent were pursuing a range of cultural and artistic activities; 80 per cent were involved in knowledge development and skills training; 73 per cent had been undertaking public education, including working with the local media; and 37 per cent were developing and operating small community-based businesses and thus involved in economic development activities.

Strategies and concepts of empowerment

In concluding this chapter we will briefly relate the different strategies that we have distinguished to the different concepts of empowerment evident within the burgeoning literature on this topic.

The varying priorities given to seeking change within the mental health system, change within the personal and social lives of those living with psychological distress and change within the broader social, economic and cultural spheres reflect the different domains within which empowerment may be sought and practised. The sphere within which there has been perhaps the least action in the UK is the socio-economic domain. Individual advocacy has taken up welfare benefits issues, but there has been little action directly addressing issues of poverty experienced by mental health service users at a collective level. A user group in Merseyside has sought to include this within their overall campaigning strategy (Davis, personal communication), but at a national level campaigning in relation to welfare benefits issues has been largely dominated by the disabled people's movement.

However, it is quite clear that the practice of empowerment collectively being pursued within the user movement in the UK and elsewhere cannot be understood solely by reference to notions of choice as a route to consumer empowerment. Whether or not the term 'citizenship' is explicit within the discourse of mental health user or survivor groups, their objectives are explicitly concerned with the relationship between people who use mental health services, the communities in which they live, and the state that defines the circumstances in which and nature of the support they receive. To this extent citizen empowerment rather than consumer empowerment should be considered a more appropriate description of the strategies being pursued.

Nevertheless, mental health policy and mental health services play a very significant part in the lives of people living with severe psychological distress. They affect people's lives directly through the part they play in defining and responding to their mental health problems, and more broadly in terms of shaping public perceptions and hence the possibilities for living in the public sphere. In view of this most sections of the mental health user movement are prepared to work within the system in order to achieve change. While there are many examples of robust challenges being offered to mental health workers, there is also a powerful stream of thought that the aim should be to transform the practice of workers, rather than to disempower them. How that might happen will be picked up again in Chapter 8.

Beyond this, some of the most significant changes that are taking place are taking place within the knowledge domain. The potentially subversive results of the insertion of users and survivors within systems of knowledge production and dissemination may be more powerful than strategies based on seeking control over service provision. Such strategies immediately raise the tensions and ambiguities inherent in the categorisation of people as 'service users'. When someone who has been an in-patient in a psychiatric hospital stands in front of a class of postgraduate students they are there as a teacher or educator, not as a user or consumer. When we as university lecturers and researchers work with people who have used services as research students or co-researchers, our relationships are defined by the supervisor–student relationship or the research team relationships. More directly, perhaps, there is growing recognition that many of those who work in the mental health services could themselves be identified as service users. While coming out in that way is still highly problematic, the NHS has been sufficiently aware of the significance of this to propose a need for research exploring the mental health of the NHS workforce.

The discomfort that is created by not being able to neatly assign people to the 'user' or 'worker' category is a useful reminder that empowerment cannot be achieved as long as it is only conceived in terms of offering choices over the nature of treatment or the location of service provision. The changes that are sought through empowerment strategies are changes in the lives of people living with severe psychological distress, changes in the nature of the mental health system which should meet their mental health needs, and changes within the society in which they live their lives as citizens.

4

Diversity, difference and empowerment

The experience of severe psychological distress is one which can come to people at any stage in their lives. It can affect people of all classes and ethnic groups. However, we cannot assume that either the issues around which different users of mental health services might wish to organise, or the processes through which they might become empowered will be the same. There are many ways of looking at this. For example, different forms of distress affect people in different ways. For some the experience of psychological distress will be of extreme depression, isolation and lethargy. Others, or the same people at other times, might experience rushes of energy which cause them to engage in constant activity and movement. Others may hear voices which act as a benign or antagonistic influence on them. The interest and ability to act to represent individual or collective interests may vary throughout the life of someone living with severe psychological distress, as will the mechanisms through which they can become empowered.

One important characteristic of the collective organisation of users of mental health service users is that individual differences can be supported and accommodated without an interruption of collective action. If someone feels unable to act as their own advocate they can seek help from a peer. If a user trainer is unwell when they are due to provide a training course, the Solihull MIND model discussed in Chapter 3 ensures that a colleague can take over that slot. But as well as individual and life course differences, there is also evidence of structural difference in the distribution of psychological distress and the way in which it is experienced between women and men, between white people and black people. There is also evidence that the way people are treated within the mental health system is affected by whether they are a man or a woman, black or white. In this chapter we consider the way in which our understanding of empowerment needs to include understanding of the particular experience of power and powerlessness according to gender and ethnicity. We will also look at the way in which women and black people have sought to develop their own, sometimes separate, ways of organising and achieving change within the mental health user movement. We will relate that to action among women and black people as part of broader social movements which seek to challenge oppression and disadvantage.

Crazy women

In languages which distinguish between male and female nouns, madness is feminine: la folie in French; la pazzia in Italian. Women, by their nature it seems, are more likely to be mad than are men. In Chapter 1 we discussed how constructions of 'the mentally disordered' as lacking autonomy and rationality can contribute to the powerlessness of people experiencing psychological distress. This operates both through the overt exercise of power over people identified as mentally disordered 'for their own good' and also by the internalisation of feelings of incompetence, lack of worth and low self-esteem.

The socially constructed nature of 'mental disorder' has a clear gender dimension. In her book *Justice Unbalanced: Gender, Psychiatry and Judicial Decisions* Allen (1987) analyses the way in which women and men who have been convicted of criminal offences and are considered to be suffering from mental disorder are treated differently by both the legal and psychiatric systems. Rather than seeking to explain why such differences in outcome should come about, Allen concentrates on seeking to understand *how* such differences arise. She concludes that the differences emerge from the intersection of two discourses: those governing the involvement of psychiatry in criminal justice, and those which structure the assessment and judgement of the offender. Both discourses are embodied in legal statutes, codes of practice and service systems as well as in the professional practice of those empowered to take decisions about psychiatric and criminal disposals. These professional and legal discourses are themselves embedded in 'common-sense' understandings and everyday attitudes. Allen notes:

> Across this broad discursive structure – unlike the other – the division by gender is both insistent and pervasive. As I have demonstrated, medico-legal discourse constructs male and female subjects in divergent terms. It cannot conceive of a subject in whom gender is not a fundamentally determining attribute, and at all levels the gender of the subject will influence the interpretation of the behaviours and the assessment of appropriate responses. Thus

materially similar events acquire different significances in the lives of male and female subjects; similar patterns of behaviour are differently interpreted as evidence of male and female personalities; and in male and female cases different criteria are called into play in assessing the 'same' parameters of legal culpability, personal pathology, and clinical need. (Allen, 1987: 113)

In practice what this means is that women who have been convicted of an imprisonable offence are more likely than men to receive 'psychiatric disposals'. Women tend to be described in psychiatric reports as passive sleepwalkers in the presence of violent and tragic events. Rather than women being considered to have committed acts of violence or criminality, such events are described as 'having occurred'. Allen offers this example from a psychiatric report on a woman accused of murder, manslaughter and arson:

I do not think it at all likely that she planned to commit this crime. The crime in all probability developed from the original fight, and the tragic events that followed were caused by Karis's dissociation from her own feelings, so that she was in an emotionless trance and unable to appreciate what she had done, or to take steps to prevent a further tragedy occurring. At this point she could not make responsible decisions. This too was her natural defence against extreme stress. It is a well known and typical hysterical reaction. (ibid.: 44)

The term 'hysterical' reveals the profoundly gendered constructs with which psychiatry works. The term comes from the Greek word for womb.

Allen's analysis provides a detailed and particular example of a more general construction of women as passive objects rather than active agents creating their own lives.

The realm of wrongdoing or deviance, as of normality, is a world in which we assume individuals to be agents: persons who are responsible for their thoughts and actions which are judged by social standards. In contrast, the realm of mental disorder is a world in which individuals are assumed to be subject to forces which they themselves cannot immediately control – they are passive rather than active. However, since assumptions or denials of agency are in practice gender-related, it follows that gender underpins the allocation of categories of problematic thought and action to the realms of mental disorder or deviance. What is typically problematic among men is more likely to be assigned to the category of wrongdoing; among women to the category of mental disorder. (Busfield, 1996: 105–6)

Passivity and powerlessness go hand in hand. Women are more likely than men to be subject to unwelcome and even coercive interventions 'for their own good'. Thus women have been more often the subject of assessments for compulsory detention under the Mental Health Act than have men and, following assessment a slightly higher proportion of women have been admitted under section (Barnes *et al.*, 1990). Ashton (1991) calculated that 66 per cent of prescriptions for psychotropic drugs go to women. Some of the reasons for this can be found in the words of a London GP talking about differences in the way he responds to women and men patients:

> Most doctors are men, most patients are women. I have no doubt that there are some paternal, protective and sexual feelings between doctors and patients that make male doctors think they must help women more [than men]. I think that women are under far more stress than men basically in a sexist society.
>
> It's also something to do with the way men present themselves. It is a sort of macho thing; they are less involving, more matter-of-fact: here's the problem and let's see what we can do about it. I feel that prescribing for men is not as urgent or so necessary. Men talk about problems in a different way. I suppose the one benefit of a macho approach to things is that they tend to say 'I don't need tablets, I can manage it myself.' (Quoted in Curran and Golombok, 1985: 54)

A rather different aspect of the way in which the gendered construction of mental illness consigns women to a passive position, unable to resist the forces which sweep away their sanity, is that which links psychiatric disorder in women with aspects of female sexuality and with the reproductive cycle. A preoccupation with women's sexual behaviour is evident in these responses from the mental health system:

> Betty is... 'promiscuous, a difficult patient whose only interest is in sex, smoking and cups of tea'. (File notes on a patient in a psychiatric hospital, 1989. From Barnes and Maple, 1992)
>
> In the past she had been at risk of going out late and chatting up men. It hasn't happened so far, but on past performance I expect it would. (Approved Social Worker notes on recommendation for compulsory detention. Quoted by Sheppard, 1990)

Women are 'at risk' from their sexuality, and if they succumb to mental disorder, then uninhibited sexual behaviour is read as a symptom of the disorder itself. That risk can be cited as a reason for involuntary detention, and as a management problem for mental health workers.

Figert (1996) explores the way in which women's 'raging hormones' have been implicated in 'crazy' behaviours which have led to the designation of pre-menstrual syndrome (PMS) as a psychiatric disorder. She quotes examples of 'jokes', cards and badges which have developed in response to the identification of PMS as a 'problem'. One example of a greeting card emphasises the stereotypical incompetence assigned to women, in particular those at the mercy of their hormones: 'Why does it take three women with PMS to change a light bulb? Answer: it just does!!'

There is a further aspect of this construction of the relationship between women's assumed lack of agency and mental disorder which is relevant to our discussion about power and powerlessness. This is the assumed 'weakness' inherent in women's self-identification based in relationships to others. Developmental psychologists have theorised the progression to maturity as a process of separation and growing independence. Feminist psychologists have developed a theory of 'self-in-relation' to emphasise that a perception of oneself as a strongly relational one is not a sign of immaturity as male psychology has sought to suggest. Rather than interpret women's desire for connectedness as weakness, Kaplan and Surrey have suggested that 'the ability to experience, comprehend and respond to the inner state of another person is a highly complex process relying on a high level of psychological development and ego strength' (1986: 82). More recently connections have been drawn between attachment theory in the context of individual psychology and social and political processes in the public sphere (Kraemer and Roberts, 1996). Far from women's personal need for connectedness being a weakness, it can be reconstructed as a source of strength in the political sphere in which the capacity for collective action among people who, individually, might have little power, is a necessary resource.

It is clear from this brief discussion of agency and mental disorder in women that 'mental health' is itself a gendered concept. If this is the case, then instruments designed to 'measure' mental disorder will measure it in a gendered way. Furthermore, if what becomes defined as mental disorder is affected by the gender of the person concerned, this will affect the number of people who become 'users' of mental health services. This makes it hard to talk about 'real differences' in the level and extent to which women and men experience psychological distress. Recent analyses of hospital admission statistics have demonstrated that the over-representation of women within the mental health system has shifted somewhat in recent times (Prior, 1999). Statistics demonstrating differences in the use of services should not, however, be confused with evidence about the prevalence of psychological distress. Intervening factors, such as the availability, accessibility and appropriateness of services, and health and illness behaviours are themselves affected by gender. Even community surveys which attempt to measure the prevalence of severe psychological distress among the general population are not unproblematic because of the gendered nature of the screening instruments used (Busfield, 1996).

Rather than enter into a discussion about the disputed evidence relating to comparative prevalence of severe psychological distress according to gender, it is perhaps more useful to look at the different circumstances of women who attract a diagnostic label and to consider how they are treated within the mental health system.

One well-known study that looked at a general population sample rather than at those already in contact with the mental health system is Brown and Harris' (1978) study in Camberwell, London. They were sufficiently convinced by previous evidence that they should only look at women in order to explore 'The Social Origins of Depression'. They found that between 20 per cent and 40 per cent of working-class women in Camberwell were identified as having psychological problems approaching the point at which a clinical diagnosis might be given.

Since Brown and Harris only looked at women they were not able to make any comparisons between the circumstances of women and men who become depressed. They started with the assumption of greater likelihood that women would experience depression and sought to identify factors that made women 'vulnerable'. Therefore they could not examine the circumstances in which men might be vulnerable to depression and whether or not these were significantly different from the circumstances associated with depression in women.

The vulnerability factors they identified were:

- not having paid employment outside the home;
- not having an intimate relationship with husband or boyfriend (they did not ask about intimate relationships with other women);
- having 3 or more children under 14 living at home;
- the early loss of a mother.

Other studies have similarly highlighted the role of women's experiences and responses to the social circumstances in which they find themselves, rather than their biology, in explaining why women are apparently more likely than men to experience severe psychological distress. Cochrane's conclusion, from his review of evidence of gender differences in the experience of mental health problems, was that differences must relate to social rather than biological factors because they were not consistent between different societies and at different times in history (Cochrane, 1983).

Jenkins (1985) sought to test out whether differences related to sex or to the different circumstances and experiences of women and men. She selected a sample of women and men in the same circumstance: direct entry civil servants on executive officer grade, aged 20–35, who had been in post for the same amount of time. She found no evidence of differences in their mental health – further evidence that a greater prevalence of psychological distress among women must relate to differences in the experiences and circumstances of women, rather than inherent vulnerability.

More recently a range of research studies have demonstrated the high likelihood that women who end up in the mental health system will have experienced physical or sexual abuse at some stage in their lives. The precise percentage of women users of mental health services who have been sexually abused is very hard to determine. Definitions of abuse vary and topics such as this are extremely difficult to research. Nonetheless a number of studies in the UK, USA, Canada and elsewhere have revealed that 50 per cent or more women in receipt of hospital-based psychiatric services have histories of abuse – demonstrating the significance of the way in which sexual power exerted over women can be implicated in subsequent severe distress (for example Bryer *et al.*, 1987; Ross *et al.*, 1989; Brown and Anderson, 1991). There is also increasing evidence of the existence of abuse within hospitals and in relationships between women and their therapists (for example Potier, 1993; Wood and Copperman, 1996). For women who have already experienced abuse, many of the 'normal practices' of psychiatry can be experienced as a repetition of abuse (Jennings, 1998). Mental health services are not immune from the often oppressive relationships which exist between men and women.

Empowerment in the case of women experiencing severe psychological distress must engage with the objective circumstances of women's lives, including the overt exercise of power represented by acts of violence and abuse. It must also address assumptions about gender roles and identity – in particular with the way in which these place women in a passive or dependent position – and with the gendered constructions of mental disorder themselves.

Women organising

Kalinowski and Penney (1998) have suggested that the 'ex-patients' movement in the USA was influenced, if not inspired, by feminist thinking and the example of the women's movement. Certainly, as in the UK, many of the key players in the movement have been and continue to be women and critiques of the discourses of professionalism owe much to feminist analyses of patriarchal power. Furthermore, methods of consciousness-raising that were developed within the women's movement to make connections between personal experience and political analysis and action have parallels within the mental health user movement. In this context consciousness raising has enabled the realisation that many of the experiences of people who have used mental health services are the result not of mental health problems per se, but of the discrimination and disadvantage that is attached to a psychiatric diagnosis.

The role of support groups in personal empowerment has been and continues to be an important one. Furthermore, personal empowerment can be an important first step to taking collective action to achieve broader change. Feminist conceptions of power and empowerment encompass not only women gaining 'power over', but also their movement into 'power to', drawing on power from within themselves to act. Thus the way in which women organise is as significant as the issue around which they take action. This has involved challenging the division of the world into separate public and private spheres and engaging with power relations in the domestic as well as the public spheres. It has also meant working in non-hierarchical groups and organisations in order to challenge the dominance and oppression that can develop within political organisations as elsewhere.

Women have been active participants in many different struggles for social change (Dominelli, 1990; Rowbotham, 1992; Lovenduski and Randall, 1993; Wainwright, 1994; Doyal, 1995; Afshar, 1998). However, the constraints on women's lives – such as poverty, isolation within the domestic sphere, responsibility for the care of children and other relatives – and the danger of public spaces can make it difficult for women to come together. Often their participation has been in the face of opposition from husbands and families because it challenges not only the gendered dynamics of family life, but also the construction of women as dependent and passive (Rowlands, 1998). While the feminist movement of the 1960s and 70s sought to organise around the shared experience and identity of 'woman', differences between women – of age, 'race', sexuality, disability, and class – surfaced to expose the racist and classist assumptions that underpinned much feminist theorising and action. For example, disabled women (Morris, 1989), lesbians and black women have found it important to organise separately sometimes in order to insert awareness of the impact of other forms of discrimination into feminist analysis and action. The women's movement has had to learn to work with difference as well as to build solidarity.

Women's health has been a particular focus for collective action among women throughout the world. During the late 1960s and 70s many women's groups focused their attention on raising women's awareness of their own bodies and on 'rediscovering' women's knowledge about self-health care, which had been hidden by the professionalisation of medicine (Ehrenreich and English, 1979). Reproductive rights issues have been a key focus for women's health politics. Campaigning in this area has engaged with women's rights to both control their own fertility and to transform the experience of childbirth (Oakley, 1980). This has had some success and has been taken up within official policy guidelines (DoH, 1993). Other women's health issues have also been the subject of collective action. For example, women's campaigns concerning breast cancer have had some success in influencing medical treatment and in raising awareness, particularly in the USA (Wilkinson and Kitzinger, 1994).

Other action has focused not on 'women's issues' per se, but has been in response to evidence and experience of gender inequalities in health and access to health services – including focusing specifically on women's experience of psychological distress.

Fighting mad

Women in the mental health users/survivors movement and their allies have highlighted differential access to certain forms of mental health service (Williams *et al.*, 1993), abuses experienced by women in the mental health system (Nilbert *et al.*, 1989; Wood and Copperman, 1996) and the gendered assumptions on which both diagnosis and treatment can be based (Williams *et al.*, 1993). They have been engaged in developing alternative models of services (Pound *et al.*, 1985; MIND, 1986; Ernst and Maguire, 1987; Good Practices in Mental Health, 1994) and alternative understandings of the origins and impact of psychological distress among women (Millett, 1991; Perkins *et al.*, 1996). In this context they have sought to give voice to the suppressed narratives of abuse which underlie the experiences of many women in the mental health system (Barnes and Maple, 1992; MIND, 1992; Simpson, 1995; Jennings, 1998). They have also engaged with disputes over diagnosis and the tendency to psychiatrise 'women's problems' (Figert, 1996) and have exposed the particular inequalities experienced by women within secure psychiatric services designed primarily around the circumstances and needs of men (Potier, 1993; Barnes, 1996; Barnes and Stephenson, 1996).

Women have been active participants in the mental health user movement at both local and national level. They have also organised separately within the movement, often in alliances between users and workers within the system. For example, both 'Women in MIND' and MIND's 'Stress on Women' project involved women who have used services working together with campaigners and mental health professionals. So did the work on 'Good Practices in Mental Health for Women', a project undertaken as a result of collaboration between GPMH and the European Regional Council of the World Federation of Mental Health. This was part of a wider European initiative intended to highlight women's experience of psychological distress and of psychiatric systems (Perkins *et al.*, 1996). Women in Special Hospitals and Secure Units (WISH) employs women who have been patients in secure hospitals, but also has mental health workers, academic and other allies as paid employees and members of an advisory board. While it would be wrong to assume an easy identity between women users and women professionals within the mental health system, or to ignore the very real differences of power which exist, many local and national initiatives have been pursued by working together. This may in part reflect common experiences. When women workers are doing their job, they are also aware of, for example, the fact that they have to pick a child up from school. Women professionals may thus be more likely to understand the way in which the complexities of women's lives can contribute to their experience of psychological distress.

Some women have put their energies into developing alternative sources of support to women in distress. For women who have experienced psychological distress the existence of safe spaces is an important part of creating the conditions within which they can become empowered. As we have seen above, entry into the mental health system cannot be equated with entering a place of safety and protection and can itself do further damage to women's sense of themselves as autonomous actors. One response to this within the user movement has been to create women-only spaces within user-run services. One example is the 'Women's Space' within one of the user-led initiatives described by Barnes *et al.* (1996). This comprises a comfortable sitting area, office and kitchen solely for the use of women. It was created in acknowledgement that sharing the identity of 'users' with men did not overcome the potential for harassment, nor for the need of women to be separate at times. For many of the women using this centre the existence of the women's space was an important motivation for their involvement in the user group as a whole. One talked of needing simply to spend time in the women's space without joining in any conversations or activities before she felt able to play a part in the group as a whole. Subsequently she produced several documents about what the group as a whole should consider doing and became an active member of the mixed space.

User groups, however, are not immune from conflicts which can develop on the lines of gender and ethnicity. Although some men in the group acknowledged a need for separate space for women, recognising that women can experience distress and harm from male mental health service users as well as from men generally, this in itself was not enough to overcome gender conflicts between members. Some men were suspicious of what went on in the women-only space and would come into the women's space, using the excuse that messages had to be delivered. One male user said 'this is a mental health project, it's not about women's issues' and quoted a recent newspaper article about an increase in suicides among young men, suggesting that the needs of men were being ignored. Other men were concerned that the women seemed to be better organised than the men, to talk more to each other and to create a more sympathetic environment. They were worried that the women's space might separate and the centre end up as two projects and that the men would miss out if women organised separately.

In another area, a woman working with a local user group talked of the way in which men always seemed to end up chairing meetings, even when it had been agreed that roles should be shared. She suggested that men were used to being in control and were frightened when they felt they did not know what was happening.

Many women-centred services developed within the voluntary sector, work on models in which the women who use the services also create them. This is part of the philosophy of NEWPIN, a national organisation with local services to support women in psychological distress who have young children. As well as providing one-to-one counselling, group therapy and workshops for women with young children, women who receive support are expected to attend a personal development programme once they are ready. New members are introduced and supported by women already using the service. Some move on from this to become co-ordinators of the service, while a regular users' meeting ensures that women users are involved in all aspects of the running of the project.

In a different way, women who have experienced self-injury and who have been through the mental health system and experienced little help from it have developed their own services. Bristol Crisis Service for Women was set up by survivors who wanted to offer an alternative to mainstream mental health services to women who self-harm. Funding shortfalls have meant that they are not able to provide the range of services they would like, but they do provide a crisis telephone line and receive calls from all round the country. The main issues they deal with are self-harm, sexual abuse, eating distress and tranquillisers.

As well as developing alternative services and systems of support, women active in the mental health user movement are also involved in trying to ensure that mainstream services more effectively respond to women's needs and circumstances. For example, women working within User Voice in South Birmingham, have taken on the issues of women in hospital who have been sexually assaulted or who spent their time in hospital in fear of such assault. They have also been concerned about how the lack of child-care facilities within local mental health services, even those which have provided women-only groups, make it impossible for women with children to use services effectively. The local mental health trust, for example, argued that a family visiting area with a play worker and toys for children was not a priority for its new psychiatric hospital and that they could not afford to develop women-only wards.

Practical action to develop alternatives or to create more women-friendly mainstream mental health services are based in an analysis of the links between psychological distress and women's lives as a whole. The outcomes of such action have enabled many women to receive support which they would not have otherwise experienced. But the significance of women's action within the mental health user movement goes beyond such important achievements. One woman activist said during a research interview:

> it's given me a life and without it I wouldn't have dreamed of doing half the things I do now. It's given me confidence, assurance... I get up now and speak

at a conference quite happily. A few years ago I would have no more done that than fly! So really we are here for ourselves as well as other people.

Demonstrating the capacity to act to create change not only has significance for the personal empowerment of individual women but also challenges the construction of women as powerless and passive. The sight of a woman user of mental health services speaking on national and international platforms about her own experiences and about ways in which services might change provides an image to counteract stereotypes of passive women, to whom things over which they have no control just happen.

Ethnic difference and mental distress

There can be no doubt that, if you are from an African-Caribbean background and living in the UK, your experience of mental health services is likely to be different from that of the white majority – you are more likely to receive hospital treatment, to be diagnosed as having a psychotic illness and to be subject to compulsory detention; less likely to receive psychotherapy; and likely to be given higher levels of medication. Differences also exist in the pattern of services received by members of other ethnic minority groups. It is important to unpack the reasons behind these differences in order to understand why black service users might bring particular perspectives to the mental health service users/survivors movement.

Hospital admission and incidence rates of distress

Precisely comparing hospital admission rates of different groups is fraught with difficulties as no national statistics are available and analyses are reliant on a series of partial and usually localised statistics. The problem with these is that they could reflect both genuine differences in need and local differences in policy and practice and cannot necessarily be taken to be nationally representative. In the Bowl and Barnes (1993) study, for example, there were large differences in the experiences of different ethnic groups in different local authority areas. There have also been difficulties in identifying base population sizes which may significantly distort comparative rates (Sashidharan, 1993).

Nonetheless, some overall patterns are detectable. McGovern and Cope (1987) and Cochrane and Bal (1989) have clearly identified that African-Caribbeans are over-represented in hospital admissions. In particular, they are three times as likely to be admitted with a first diagnosis of schizophrenia (King *et al.*, 1994; Van Os *et al.*, 1996). Evidence about South Asian groups suggests similar or slightly higher rates of admission with psychosis than those for the general population (Cochrane and Bal, 1989; King *et al.*, 1994). Both these broad groups are less likely to be admitted with depression, however (Cochrane and Bal, 1989). More recent enquiry has also suggested important differences between different South Asian sub-groups, for example, between those of Bangladeshi and Indian origin, and between those new to the UK and those who were born here or entered the UK before the age of eleven (Nazroo, 1997).

Of course, hospital use is only one indicator of the incidence and effect of mental distress. Studies which have shown all contact with psychiatric services show a similar picture and one study of such contact claims to show that the incidence rate of schizophrenia within the African-Caribbean population is as much as thirteen times higher than that of the general population (Harrison *et al.*, 1988), although considerable doubts remain about the robustness of the research (Sashidharan and Francis, 1993). Equally significantly, such figures are not figures of the incidence of mental distress in the community. They have been mediated by an interaction with health services and as such will also reflect *inter alia* the willingness of members of different groups to present themselves for a service; their ability to convey a need for particular forms of help; the interpretation of relatively unskilled personnel in primary care or casualty departments that further specialist help is required; and the propensity of a variety of other agents such as the police, the courts and the general public to refer members of different groups for unsolicited intervention. Yet these figures are not without value, not least because a comparison of service use figures with general population incidence figures can reveal something of how mental health services respond to members of different ethnic groups.

The most comprehensive attempt to measure the incidence of mental distress among members of ethnic minority groups formed part of the Fourth National Survey of Ethnic Minorities. While this confirmed slightly higher rates of non-affective psychosis among African-Caribbeans, the difference was much smaller than indicated by the treatment statistics and indeed not statistically significant (Nazroo, 1997).

Furthermore the difference is accounted for almost entirely by women, with no discernible difference between African-Caribbean and white men. The study also showed a rate of depression among the African-Caribbean group that was 60 per cent higher than that for the white population – twice as high for African-Caribbean men. Rates of non-affective psychosis among the South Asian groups were either slightly (or in the case of Bangladeshis substantially) below those of the white population. All of the South Asian groups had lower rates of depression but there were significant differences between migrants and non-migrants which may reflect problems of using standard instruments for identifying psychiatric illness, particularly depression, in a cross-cultural context (Kleinman, 1987; Jadhav, 1996). Certainly rates of both depression and psychosis for non-migrant South Asians in this study were remarkably similar to those for the white population.

Different colour, different treatment

In understanding the way black people experience mental health services, particular significance attaches to how they come to receive hospital treatment. While most patients are admitted to psychiatric hospital as informal patients, some black people are much more likely to be there because of the application of compulsion. Bowl and Barnes (1993) show that people from African-Caribbean backgrounds are referred for assessment for civil compulsory admission at a rate of 204 per 100,000 population (compared to 117 per 100,000 for the population as a whole) and are significantly more likely to be detained as a result. Similarly, black people are much more likely to be subjected to some form of forensic psychiatry (McGovern and Cope, 1987; Cope, 1989) and are over-represented in special hospitals (Norris, 1984). Other research has shown black defendants in court are less likely to be given bail and are more likely to be given orders for compulsory treatment (Browne, 1990).

Research has also suggested that section 136, which allows the police to remove people from public places if they believe them to be mentally disordered and either their own health and safety is at risk or they pose a threat to public order, sees the removal of African-Caribbeans off the streets at 2½ times the rate of white people (Bean *et al.*, 1991).

In contrast to this evidence of over-representation among those receiving the most restrictive forms of support and control, there is evidence that black people are under-represented within out-patient services (Littlewood and Cross, 1980), self-referred services (Frederick, 1991) and day centres. They may also be receiving less help for their mental distress from GPs. Although just as likely as other groups to report these difficulties to their GPs, for example, African-Caribbeans are much less likely to receive medication for psychosis or depression. Members of South Asian groups are also less likely to be treated with anti-depressants or minor tranquillisers, although more likely to be prescribed major tranquillisers when experiencing psychosis (Nazroo, 1997).

Within hospitals, black people also experience different treatment – for example, more often being placed in locked wards (Bolton, 1984). African-Caribbeans are also over-represented in secure units (Jones and Berry, 1986), more likely to receive physical treatments, including electro-convulsive therapy (ECT), than whites (Littlewood and Cross, 1980) and are less likely to receive talking treatments (McKenzie *et al.*, 1995). Furthermore fears that some treatments may be used inappropriately because of their effect in pacifying black patients are lent support by the finding that 39 per cent of black patients receiving ECT do not have a diagnosis of depression as opposed to 16 per cent of white patients. African-Caribbeans are also more likely to receive major tranquillisers and intramuscular medication (Chen *et al.*, 1991) and, indeed, heavier doses of medication. Some research also suggests that ECT is over-used with people of Asian origin (Shaikh, 1985).

Explanations of ethnic difference

It is possible to identify five broad strands of explanation for these clear differences in experience:

- the 'ethnic vulnerability' hypothesis;
- the 'migration' hypothesis;
- problems of accurate measurement;
- problems with the very nature of psychiatric assessment;
- issues of racism within the mental health system and particularly institutional racism.

The ethnic vulnerability hypothesis suggests that members of some groups are particularly vulnerable to mental ill health. Sometimes, notwithstanding the clear refutation of the validity of the idea of distinct biological races, this takes the form of trying to isolate some biological 'weakness' among black groups that makes them more vulnerable to particular forms of distress (Fernando, 1991). Perhaps reflecting the failure to find such a link, but in keeping with a tradition of trying to locate the root of the problem within ethnic minority groups themselves rather than examine critically the framework through which distress and its roots are viewed, the focus has switched to socio-cultural explanations. One argument is that higher rates of diagnosis reflect the greater stress experienced by black people in the UK. Clearly there are groups within the black population who do suffer particular social deprivation, unemployment, racial harassment and discrimination, all of which potentially may have a negative effect on their mental health (Westwood, 1989; Skellington and Morris, 1996). Circumstances which might be seen in this way include the under-valuing of the skills and attributes of black jobseekers which leads to black workers consistently accepting less prestigious and rewarding jobs than their qualities merit; growing up in an environment with few positive black images and where negative black images abound within society; and the internal conflict and confusion that may arise from the differences between the messages they receive from their parents and from the predominant British white culture. It has particularly been suggested that Asian women can find themselves in a confusing position where cultures pull them in different directions and this could lead them to being particularly vulnerable (Soni Raleigh and Balarajan, 1992).

Our own view is that the greater incidence of stress, associated with poor social and environmental conditions and racism, should not be ignored, particularly not its role in the experiences of particular individuals when they seek explanation of and help with mental distress. However, it a weak explanatory argument for the differences in measured incidence rates of distress. The most significant objection centres on the finding that among Asian groups, who experience similar socio-economic conditions and often live in the same areas as African-Caribbeans, very different patterns of mental distress have been found. In particular those experiencing the poorest conditions – Bangladeshis – have the lowest incidence of measured mental distress (Nazroo, 1997). This leads to a further version of ethnic vulnerability – the idea that it is the variable ability of different communities to mediate the effects of stress that determines, at least in part, different incidence rates of mental distress. Hence, it is argued that some Asian populations might have a particular psychological robustness or possess certain attitudes towards mental distress that make it less likely that they will be drawn to the attention of psychiatric services and/or that the mental distress that they do experience is dealt with in different ways. There is little direct evidence of this and it would be difficult to separate any such effect from a predisposition on the part of professionals to assume that members of Asian populations do have other ways of coping and therefore not make other services available to them. It may also be, because of prior experience of inappropriate services, that members of some groups are not enthusiastic to approach mental health services because they do not think that they will get appropriate treatment. The dynamics behind such a proposition are complex, however, as a reluctance to seek help early on may be as likely to be reflected in higher final incidence rates of psychological distress as lower. What this does, however, point to is the need to understand how that complex interaction between the experience and reporting of distress and the way in which mental health services respond impacts upon different incidence rates of distress and indeed different forms of treatment. Certainly such an approach is going to be of more direct relevance to black service users than explanations that rest upon judgements about culturally-based differences in propensities to provide support or in behaviour likely to exacerbate or ameliorate distress. These may, like the now largely discredited ideas about biological differences between races, simply reinforce stereotypes (Sashidharan, 1993) and discourage the careful investigation of the particular circumstances of individuals presenting for assistance with severe psychological distress.

The migration/selection hypothesis is a related set of ideas often offered to explain the under-representation of Asian populations in studies of the incidence of distress. This proposes that stronger people (genetically, biologically and/or who are more socially adaptive) may be selected for migration and that, therefore, those that have come to the UK are likely to be more resistant to the concomitant pressures. While such an explanation might be consistent with lower rates of reported distress among some Asian groups it does not fit easily with the much higher rates recorded among the African-Caribbean population, nor does it help explain the differences in diagnosis between groups. Neither is it consistent with the finding that non-migrant members of the same South Asian groups show similar rates of incidence to the UK's white population (Nazroo, 1997). Instead Nazroo suggests that apparent lower rates of incidence of poor mental health are strongly influenced by the difficulties that relative newcomers have in getting to know how the system here works and expressing themselves in ways which will be picked up by European psychiatric medicine.

Diagnosis, mis-diagnosis and racism

There are, of course, very real problems in consistently measuring the incidence of psychological distress, particularly in a multi-cultural context. The methodology of the study by Harrison *et al.* (1988), which showed such high rates of schizophrenia among African-Caribbeans, has attracted considerable criticism (Sashidharan and Francis, 1993) including that of the vulnerability of its high rates of incidence to small changes in the classification procedures. It is also true that the most significant study based on a community sample and not relying on those already in touch with services revealed very different rates of incidence – for example, showing no excessive rates of psychosis among African-Caribbean men and significantly higher rates of (largely untreated) depression (Nazroo, 1997).

Some writers have focused upon this as a problem of 'misdiagnosis' and argued that the ethnocentric views of psychiatrists have resulted in the mis-attribution of labels such as schizophrenia (Littlewood, 1992). The common practice in the 1970s and 80s of diagnosing young black men as suffering from 'cannabis psychosis', a diagnosis hardly ever applied to anyone who was white, is often highlighted as the most extreme example of this phenomenon. A further point in support of the idea of misdiagnosis is that that black service users have their diagnoses changed frequently over time or more often than their white equivalents (Pilgrim and Rogers, 1999).

Such an analysis implies that applying higher standards in the diagnostic process would 'improve' the diagnosis of black service users (and probably reduce to a degree their tendency to be diagnosed as psychotic). A different argument is to see the differential patterns of diagnosis among different ethnic groups as not so much 'misdiagnosis' as an inevitable consequence of the reliance of psychiatric diagnosis on judgements about behaviour. Attributing to individuals, diagnostic categories, rests on identifying particular patterns of 'abnormal' behaviour or 'extraordinary' behaviour. Inevitably judgements about behaviours that are outside the norm reflect the traditions and standards of the culture in which psychiatry evolved and those whose behaviour reflects other traditions and standards are nonetheless judged by that dominant white European culture. Those whose background means they are more verbally expressive and loud, those who are more introspective and those whose spiritual understanding leads to a belief in a more direct communication with their deity or ancestors, for example, may all be vulnerable to having behaviour, seen within their own culture as acceptable, seen by western mental health professionals as indicative of severe psychological distress or madness.

Nor is this the only sense in which psychiatry cannot be culture free – 'Political, social and ideological pressures current in society always impinge on the diagnostic process by influencing questions of intelligibility, common sense, clinical opinion, pragmatism and tradition' (Fernando, 1991: 37). In particular, the process of the diagnostic interview depends on the ability and willingness of the service user to communicate what is happening to them in ways which are understandable within the framework of the dominant cultural understanding of distress. Yet our communication of feelings and experiences, like depression and hallucination, depend largely on idiomatic representation which varies greatly across cultures. Some writers have argued that the inability of western clinicians to connect with certain idioms explains in part the low rates of depression among many black groups (Krause, 1989; Fenton and Sadiq-Sangster, 1996). Similarly the importance of a particular feeling or emotion will vary according to its cultural context and, where there is a large gap in understanding between therapist/assessor and service user, this creates great potential for misunderstanding the significance of what is conveyed in a diagnostic interview. There are clear parallels here with the arguments we have made about the experience of women service users.

The reliance of psychiatry on judgements about inappropriate or abnormal behaviour would be problematic in any multi-cultural context but it attains special significance because of the role of racism. Racism within society generally may expose black people more to the stresses underpinning many experiences of distress as outlined above. It may also explain why more referrals of black people for assessment for compulsory detention come via the police (Barnes *et al.*, 1990). The inclination of the public appears to be to report black people to the police rather than to a caring service, reflecting perceptions of their potential dangerousness. Such attitudes must also be reflected in the attitudes of public servants and in the policies set out for them to follow. Hence a tendency to interpret black people's behaviour as more threatening may explain in part the propensity of the police to use section 136 more often to remove them from the streets. Certainly Browne (1990) links the high rate of psychiatric referrals from the courts to magistrates' elevated perceptions of dangerousness among this group.

It is within the psychiatric system itself that we see the most pervasive impact of racism, however, and it operates at many levels. Western psychiatry came of age as a discipline at the time when scientific racism was at its most influential and inevitably this has been reflected in its development – 'the history of psychiatry... shows the discipline to have developed as a social entity within a particular cultural tradition imbued with the racism characteristic of that tradition' (Fernando, 1991: 59). The search for biological differences to explain ethnic variations in patterns of distress reflects that history and, while this has been largely replaced by a search for cultural explanations, these remain focused upon ethnic minorities themselves rather than the context through which they are viewed. This may give rise to an element of self-fulfilling prophecy in reported distress rates. Pilgrim and Rogers (1993), for example, make the point that because there are higher rates of identification of certain diagnoses among particular ethnic minority groups, this in a circular way may lead to a predisposition to interpret the behaviour of members of those groups as signs of insanity.

The continuing perception of black people as more 'dangerous', which underpins the more custodial and restrictive treatment outlined above, may also reflect racist notions of their behaviour as more 'primitive and barbaric'. Some have suggested this treatment simply reflects their being more ill. However, there is evidence from official hospital inquiries – for example the Orville Blackwood Inquiry (SHSA, 1993) – that this treatment is often a response to assumptions about black people being more violent or more dangerous, more in need of control. Harrison *et al.* (1989) have shown how staff were more likely to be concerned about potential dangerousness of black patients after admission, despite there being no evidence of any greater aggression or violence leading to admission. Similarly, fear of violence was identified by Approved Social Workers as a critical influence when Bowl and Barnes (1993) examined their explanations for why it was more likely that a black person was detained than a white person in similar circumstances, following their assessment. Noble and Rodger (1989) also showed how non-violent African-Caribbean patients were more likely to be detained formally on a locked ward than similar white patients and that African-Caribbean patients were more likely to be reported as being violent. Commenting on this, Pilgrim and Rogers (1999) suggest that there may be in effect a spiral of violence happening here – viz. black patients are seen as being more violent and treated more coercively and so they react to this discriminatory regime in an aggressive way. That in turn makes staff become more coercive and the cycle starts again.

This itself links to another aspect of the racism that pervades the psychiatric system – the tendency to adopt a 'colour-blind approach'. In claiming to treat everybody as the same, this could be seen as a counter to the impact of stereotyping. In reality, such an approach is actually another form of discriminatory practice. Two examples will illustrate the point. Psychiatric diagnosis and treatment depend on the interpretation of behaviour. The life of black service users may well have been an experience of racism and disadvantage and prejudice because they have a mental health problem. They may also be aware of the apparent over-use of restraint and physical treatments and inevitably distrust what might happen to them in hospital. The cumulative effect may be to increase levels of fear and possibly engender an aggressive response. Both may be seen as symptoms of mental disorder. Yet to act upon them without taking into account the role of the very particular experiences of the patient being assessed, in this case those aspects of their experience based upon their ethnic background, would inevitably be misleading. Similarly black service users aware of the use of coercion, or cynical about the insensitivity of services to their needs, may be reluctant to engage and this in turn may be read as a lack of co-operation. In each case, treating patients as the same may disadvantage black patients leading to an inappropriate diagnosis and treatment regime. Treating people equally in contrast implies recognising and taking into account the impact of their ethnic background.

Fernando (1991) puts the argument about racism into a broader context. He sees western psychiatry as having achieved ascendancy over the psychiatric traditions of other cultures and that this is based upon racist assumptions about the superiority of European modes of thought and analysis. While cross-cultural comparison is difficult, not least because it is nearly always carried out by within the context of western frameworks of understanding, it does not support the assumption of the superiority of the western system. Schizophrenia as a concept, for example, has been shown to have little predictive value as prognosis in a world context. There is also some evidence for the superiority of techniques other than those adopted by western psychiatry in relieving the distress identified in this way. Fernando's concern is with the imposition of this belief system on other cultures both here and in other parts of the world. Certainly its imposition upon those with different belief systems is potentially destructive. Intervention based on the medicalisation of distress as an illness may not only undermine the understanding of black service users but it may directly interfere with healing strategies embedded in other systems of belief. Fernando does not seek to eliminate western psychiatry, which he recognises has certain strengths.

Rather he wishes to challenge its culture bound roots underpinned by racist beliefs and create an adaptive psychiatry that recognises the validity of different belief systems and that accepts people's different cultures on equal terms.

Pilgrim and Rogers (1999) also provide another layer of over-arching explanation based upon an analysis of the discourse of psychiatry and the work of writers like Foucault (1965) and Paul Gilroy (1987). This highlights psychiatry's reliance on locating madness as essentially 'other' – as part of a process of distancing 'reason' from 'unreason', 'civilisation' from 'barbarism' (literally during the Victorian period). This has parallels in the 'new racism' that has stimulated a search for new scapegoats (for national decline and social disorder) and a redefinition of the notion of 'other' as opposed to ourselves. This in turn is linked to who is included and excluded from the main stream of society. One form of exclusion is to be defined as essentially different because of behaviour outside the norm, as happens to people diagnosed as experiencing schizophrenia. There may well, therefore, be links between exclusion because of race and because of mental health problems – they may well reinforce each other.

Within this context psychiatry can be seen as operating, in co-operation with the other wider oppressive state apparatuses, as a post-colonial Europeanised alternative to repatriation. People can still be banished but the banishment can take place not to another country but within psychiatric hospitals, reinforced by prison and physical treatments. An interesting footnote to this is that this discourse focuses strongly on the threat that people represent – not the distress they are suffering. This in turn is reflected in the relative neglect of concern about other aspects of the experience of black people, such the sadness and despair experienced by Asian women (Beliappa, 1991).

Black service users and the user movement

Given these arguments about the particular experiences of black service users, it is perhaps striking on contact with service user movement organisations that there are so few black faces.

> Black communities, specifically those of African-Caribbean and Asian origin... have not, on the whole, been involved in the movement's campaigning. (Sassoon and Lindow, 1995: 89)

It is a phenomenon also identified in writings about the service user movement in the USA (Watkins and Callicutt, 1997). Indeed, not only are black service users not strongly represented in the established UK users/survivors movement, but there is also only limited evidence of independent activity by groups of black service users.

Why is this, given the significance of the particular issues facing black service users? Part of the answer may lie with the composition of existing service user groups. First there is little reason to assume that such a diverse movement will not reflect the attitudes abroad within society generally, including the existence of direct racism. One writer from the Leicester Black Mental Health Group reflects on relationships with their fellow service users: ' I found the patients even more racist than the staff. One of them had the habit of calling me Sambo. I couldn't believe it, even mad people hate us' (Westwood *et al.*, 1989). Given their own experience of oppression, many service user groups are aware of this and some have tried to address it by undertaking anti-racist training and adopting specific anti-racist policies. Even in this context, however, there remain significant differences in understanding and interests that may inhibit black service users' participation in movement organisations. It would be too simplistic to suggest that their patient status was at the core of white services users' identities. They are also, for example, men and women, workers or parents. However, as we identify in Chapter 5, involvement in the movement and the sense of achievement and mutual support it can bring, certainly suggests that for many an identity as a service user challenging the system is more important to them than their whiteness. In contrast for many black people, given their everyday experience of racism 'Blackness is as much part of the individual as their gender. As such it may be a minor or major factor in their problem. It cannot be ignored' (Moodley, 1995: 123).

Hence, while white service users may well have sympathy with black service users because of their experience of unequal treatment within the system, the perception of many is that racism constitutes an additional factor compounding black service users' experience of mental health services. For black service users it may be more fundamental – 'Racism is thus experienced not as an additional problem but an interpretative schema through which all problems are to be understood' (Sadhoo, quoted in Sassoon and Lindow, 1995: 93). The pervasive impact of this interpretive schema on black service users' experience of distress and the responses of mental health services is clearly illustrated in the analysis above. Ignoring such differences and placing too much stress on the shared experiences of services may, therefore, simply serve to alienate black service users.

Differences in the concerns of black and white service users are also revealed in quite pragmatic forms. Moodley (1995) reports on a user survey that, while showing some congruence in their concerns, also revealed the greater importance black service users attached to the availability of staff of their own colour and help with finding jobs. It also showed them to be less happy about the information they received about diagnosis and treatments.

There may be other deterrents to activism by black service users. We reflect in Chapter 5 that activism may be problematic for all service users where it involves exposure of differences with those providing a service on which they depend. The experience of African-Caribbean service users of higher dosages of medication and more frequent resort to compulsion, as well as their experience of power exercised in other aspects of their lives, may well inhibit participation in hospital-based groups. Users of Asian origin may not have confidence that they will be able to communicate easily or fear that their culture will be misrepresented or subject to disapprobation. Further, while identity as an activist can bring respect to service users, in some cultural contexts the identity of mental health service user itself may become an added threat to an already vulnerable status and lead to a loss of respect within a service users' own community (Sassoon and Lindow, 1995). This in turn would be a deterrent to continuing association with mental health services on discharge from hospital and a disincentive to activism. Even the strategies of empowerment that focus on enhancing the individual's control over their own environment may clash with the fundamental beliefs of those from a collectivist culture wrestling to come to terms with distress within the context of a different set of cultural explanations.

The effect of these differences may also be reflected in different organisational responses to perceived problems with the mental health services. The campaign around the case of Orville Blackwood, a young black man who died in Broadmoor High Security Hospital provides an illustration. The campaign owed much to the energy of Orville's mother but was also well supported by black mental health professionals and black figures from the media and other walks of life. It further had a focus that went broader than simply the particular oppression faced by black people in the psychiatric system. It was also set within the context of black people's experience of other forms of coercion and manifestations of racism. The appeal to black workers from both within and without the system may also have reflected a direct relationship between the negative images of black people within the psychiatric system and how black people in general are perceived. As such the mutual experience of being black in a racist society would have more resonance and give rise to a greater sense of solidarity in resistance than a shared experience of the use of mental health services. Sassoon and Lindow (1995) argue that there has been a similar convergence in the interests of black service users and black workers and service organisations in campaigning against the over-diagnosis of schizophrenia and other issues impacting upon black service users.

Nonetheless it should not be assumed that black workers and advocacy groups can fully represent the perspectives of service users – theirs remains a different experience. It is also true that black workers predominantly receive the same training and orientation and share many of the same interests as other workers. Inevitably, therefore, there have begun to emerge support groups of black service users such as the groups for Somali women experiencing emotional distress in Sheffield discussed in Chapter 3, although many retain strong links with black advocacy groups. Sassoon and Lindow (1995) describe the example of the Black Carers and Clients Project which is located at the Afro-Caribbean Mental Health Project in Brixton, London. While its strategies have a central focus on developing an understanding of the impact of racism and place importance on education and training of professionals and policy makers, it has also given rise to the development of individual support groups. Awaaz – a group for Asian service users in North Manchester – similarly has a commitment to trying to influence mainstream services but also gives weight to the direct provision of culturally appropriate support which those mainstream services still fail to deliver.

This in turn provides a pointer to what might be seen as two related but distinct dimensions to the strategies adopted by black service users groups. They are engaged in campaigning to establish equal treatment within mental health services. They also provide a base from which black service users can explore what is needed to develop more helpful and appropriate responses to distress, sometimes rooted in revisiting views of healing from their own traditions, that are more appropriate to their specific needs.

As these strategies develop and proliferate, our expectation is that they will bring fresh perspectives that enrich the varied contribution of the service user movement in much the way that women organising within the movement have done.

5

Changing lives and minds

We have described in earlier chapters the gradual acceptance of the validity of the users of mental health services exercising more autonomy, either outside or inside mainstream services. We have also stressed important differences between autonomous action, initiated and controlled by people who identify themselves as users or survivors and action taken from within service systems to consult or more actively involve users in decision-making processes. In the latter context, we have described how 'benefits', whether to service users themselves or to the services, are imputed rather than always carefully thought out. In particular, confusion may arise between seeing user involvement as a therapeutic goal and creating opportunities for service users to significantly influence the nature of support provided for them.

This chapter attempts to pull together evidence, first, of the impact of user involvement on service users themselves and then on the perceptions that lay people and professionals have of service users.

Evaluating the impact of involvement strategies

How might the impact of user involvement on individual service users be evaluated? If the conventions for assessing the value of psychiatric intervention were followed, this would need to be based around a randomly controlled trial and measures that reflected the key targets of intervention within the medical discourse – there would be a focus on the reduction of symptoms. Hence, depending on the particular diagnosis, the impact of user involvement upon experience of hallucinations, delusions, feelings of worthlessness, manifestations of anger, self-neglect and self-harm, among others, would be measured. Proxy measures taken to be indicators of these reductions such as the number of admissions or days spent in hospital might also be employed. A commitment to a more community focused rehabilitation model might also lead to the inclusion of slightly different indicators such as, for example, adaptation to symptoms, ability to manage them independently in the community, lack of dependency on particular services, fewer out-patient visits.

Here is not the place to provide a detailed critique of reliance on such focused randomly controlled trials (Pilgrim, 1997b neatly summarises some of the difficulties). Nonetheless, it is fair to say that while service users themselves might well value a reduction in symptoms and a reduction in service reliance, one of the key lessons to emerge from the extension of the service users' voice is that these are not necessarily where they place most priority. Many service users see these as but side issues to their 'real' problems which they locate as being able to participate in society, support themselves and to enjoy feelings of wellbeing. Hence, many users of mental health services see their principal needs much as others do – they would value employment, a decent income, decent housing and a chance to make and sustain social relationships. These and symptom reduction are not always mutually exclusive but they may conflict.

We are reminded of a young male long-term service user with a diagnosis of schizophrenia whose life had been extremely disrupted by his experience of hallucinations and 'thought disorder'. As a consequence he was placed on medication which effectively controlled these symptoms and permitted him to live in the community. This gave him the chance to make relationships and in time he met a young woman and found his first potential partner. This had a very positive impact and brought real quality to his life. However, a side-effect of his medication was that, at least temporarily, he was impotent and eventually this became too big an impediment to the development of the relationship and it was lost. He was devastated and his quality of life nose-dived. Yet his symptoms continued to be controlled – the impact of the psychiatric intervention would register as positive within a conventional randomly controlled trial.

More significantly, of course, user involvement is not a clinical intervention technique. Indeed while it may produce therapeutic gains and be encouraged for that reason by some clinicians, and more particularly by other therapists informed by a more social paradigm, it is largely outside of their control. Indeed symptom reduction among those who become involved is rarely an explicit goal of autonomous action, as we outlined in Chapter 3. Much of the action being taken by autonomous user groups is directed outwards – either towards the mental health system and changes to be achieved in the services and policies which affect the lives of people when they are in this system, or towards society in general, to impact upon both attitudes and behaviours which further contribute to the exclusion and stigmatisation of those experiencing psychological distress (Barnes and Shardlow, 1997).

Nonetheless it is useful to reflect on what evidence there is of the impact of user involvement on individuals' clinical symptoms and on their sense of self, self-confidence and self-esteem, as well as their evaluations of its impact on their lives more broadly.

Consultation and participation – therapeutic or democratic goals?

Here it may be analytically useful to consider the impact of different forms of user action, taking first the different forms of involvement generated from within the system that were outlined in Chapter 2. The confusion between therapeutic goals and democratic goals is most apparent in the context of 'consultation' or 'participation'. A recent survey of human service organisations in the USA (covering a wider range of practice areas than mental health) committed to 'empowerment' practice gives an interesting insight into practitioner goals (Gutierrez *et al.*, 1995). Broadly, practitioners in these organisations had goals of enhancing individuals' awareness of their own strengths and building upon them – extending confidence and an ability to recognise their own power; encouraging them to exercise choice and act with autonomy; and facilitating a sense of and ability to take control over their own lives. McLean similarly notes that 'Most provider-run programs that claim to follow an "empowerment" model or service approach are likely to emphasise the client's mastery of specific social and/or occupational skills so the consumer can better adapt to an already given, uncontested social world' (McLean, 1995: 1057).

Such an approach might suggest a concern with developing service users' abilities to exercise the 'power to'. However, there is little sense here of importance being attached to successfully opening up opportunities for service users to effectively shape even that limited part of their social world with which practitioners are directly concerned. Rather there appears to be a central focus on therapeutic outcomes for the individual and indeed to see empowerment as very much an intervention technique – something professionals 'do' with their clients. In this context, collaborative involvement in their own treatment plans and broader consultations are seen as a method, alongside education and having an orientation in one-to-one work on the individual's strengths, that is useful in achieving the desired psychological growth. Inevitably there is a recognition that this can be achieved through interaction with other individuals but even here it is stressed how the work in such settings can usefully be guided by the professional worker (Caron and Bergeron, 1995).

There is little sense here of empowerment having a focus on creating social or political change, of user involvement producing longer term changes in the environment with which the individuals interact. Hence participation itself becomes a goal and whether or not it achieves anything for the individuals and their peers in terms of wider change is a less important consideration. The democratic and philosophical goals of user involvement are seen as of secondary importance. It seems unlikely that service users who have often had to steel themselves to taking part in participative arenas, of which they had little prior knowledge and which perhaps they perceived as intimidating, will have shared those views.

Consultation and participation within service establishments and their influence on service users

The frustrations that confusion over the purpose of consultation and participation can bring were highlighted in one of our own studies of user involvement in day centres and residential establishments for those experiencing mental distress in three local authorities in the UK (Bowl and Ross, 1994). The main forum for service users collectively to influence decisions in this context was the 'user committee' which had many forms and functions. Although some user committees exercised minor budgetary power, taking responsibility for managing a small element of the centre's activities such as a snack bar, most served as a consultative forum, considering mainly domestic issues such as the price of lunchtime sandwiches or the lateness of centre transport.

Indeed the function of many user committees seemed to be to provide a conduit through which to pass information from the staff to users with few formal channels of communication in the other direction. Even where a staff member facilitated a group, for example, they rarely had a formal responsibility to report back on the outcome of discussions. In this way user committees were often not fully incorporated into the structure or culture of their centres; their discussions did not inform centre policy in ways which were formally recognised nor did their concerns reach the wider audience of practitioners and decision makers in their organisations. Nonetheless, some user committees felt that they were capable of taking on more responsibility, finding ways in which the service could respond more appropriately to their needs. One committee identified, for example, how they would like to provide a drop-in service at their centre, set up and 'staffed' by members themselves.

Another indication that raises questions about perceptions of the purpose of such involvement concerns the relationship between committee members and those they 'represented'. Some committee members were nominated by staff. Others put themselves forward and found they were 'elected' as they were the only ones nominated. The method of 'election', however, is hardly the key determinant of the degree to which user committees were genuinely offering participation to service users. More significantly few user committees made use of mechanisms for noting the results of their deliberations such as minutes and there were few systematic efforts made to inform the wider user group of decisions taken during committee meetings. Nor were there systematic attempts by representatives to find out what their peers wished the user committee to do on their behalf.

In this context it appears the main benefit of user committees must be seen in terms of the individual development that might be experienced by those participating. Given our speculations about possible differences between service users and staff it is interesting to note the extent to which service users felt empowered by the experience.

Many users felt that they were often 'allowed', through their membership of user committees, to have a say in small things, such as the destination of a day trip, as a way of pretending they had some power but that when it came to 'real' issues like staffing levels they weren't deemed competent to participate. As a result, and given the negative experiences of many service users when speaking out, their desire to be involved in 'yet another committee that does nothing' diminished. Effectively such structures, where limits to the scope of service user action are carefully set out and controlled by professionals in this way, however well-intentioned and despite the benefits experienced by particular individuals, may actually be experienced as disempowering. This is because they highlight for service users the restrictions placed upon their freedom of action and effort and the limits to what they can achieve. It is also true that some other users, not on user committees, expressed concern over how decisions were made, particularly when they are taken by the user committee without what is considered 'proper' consultation with the rest of the user group, or when the committee was seen as simply a talking shop or in the pocket of the manager. The existence of a committee was not therefore particularly empowering to other members of their centre.

The effect of wider consultation and participation strategies

Within the same study we also looked at involvement in wider decision-making within the three authorities central to the study. Only one had allocated places on local joint social services and health authority planning teams for mental health services to individual representatives of service users. Within two of the authorities there were also active independent mental health service users' forums and forum members had been asked to consult on the authorities' community care plans, although they were unclear as to how far their views had influenced the final documents. Despite this, none of the service users interviewed had seen their community care plan or been consulted on its content. None, indeed were aware of their 'rights' under the community care legislation but equally, few believed that even if they had been consulted, that anyone would have taken any notice. Stating that the opportunity for consultation exists for users was seen to be of very little use unless appropriate strategies are developed which enable users to make a meaningful contribution.

Nonetheless several users from mental health centres did participate in external forums such as housing committees, sometimes in pairs, and felt that they were listened to and taken seriously. While they were not sure whether they could make material changes in service provision, they felt that they had already changed individual officers' perceptions of service users simply by attending meetings and raising the issues of concern which service users identify for themselves. The insistence by user representatives that officers explain jargon had also meant that many ideas had been simplified which had benefited other, non-user, committee members as well as their peers. Users who attended committees also talked about feeding back to their user colleagues the likely impact of the relatively abstract decisions which committees make and highlighting the lack of congruence between the priorities of the service providers and the people who are on the receiving end.

While it was clear that these individual service users did gain in terms of their perceptions of their own competence and confidence – several reported the contrast between their nervousness on first attending such meetings and their subsequent relative comfort, for example – they also reported similar frustrations to those experienced by members of centre user committees.

There was a feeling among some users that consultation and participation is never on their own terms but that they are expected to fit into the existing organisational culture of the traditional mental health agencies where formally structured meetings are held during work hours, around a 52-place table. Lord *et al.* (1998), in describing the role of service users in a process of change within a mental health organisation, stress the initial difficulties service users faced in adapting to simply sitting round a table for long periods of time. Why should it be assumed that users should fit into the structures that have evolved to suit full-time officers and party politicians? Traditional committee structures can be intimidating and complex, even for people experienced in committee work, and many of the difficulties facing service user participants could be avoided or minimised. Several users believed that if agencies were serious about consultation and participation in wider arenas, then even the format of that involvement itself should reflect the different needs of service users. For example, a number of service users work during the day and so cannot attend daytime meetings. In addition, being forced to fit into the existing committee structures means that service users and carers are always in the minority and disadvantaged by their lack of knowledge of committee protocols and access to the informal but crucial network system that underpins committee work.

The response of the Nottingham Advocacy Group has been to develop a structure which reflects service organisation in order to enable direct participation at different levels and locations within the mental health services of the city. Their relationships with local service providers are well-established and attract a considerable degree of favourable comment from officials, but activists are well aware of the way in which the rules of participation are determined by officials who still hold the power. They reported a sense of fragility in their position which can have damaging impact on people who may experience fluctuations in their mental health (Barnes *et al.*, 1999a).

Church (1996) argues that adherence to established forms within consultation exercises serves to maintain existing power differences – 'dominant groups maintain their position by teaching subordinate groups codes of behaviour such as "reason" or "politeness" which sublimate anger, for example, into non-political forms of action' (Church, 1996: 39).

Transgression of these 'rules' by service users in her study of consultation in Ontario was consistently represented by administrators and practitioners as 'bad manners', while survivors 'considered it rude for professionals/bureaucrats to expect partnership from them when meetings were hosted in environments which were not survivor-friendly, on topics which were not survivor-generated, using documents and language which were not survivor-accessible' (ibid.: 40). Some groups of users of the centres in our study (Bowl and Ross, 1994) had attempted to confront the issue of control over the form of consultation by inviting local Social Services Department officers to talk with them on their own ground, that is, at the day centres which they attended, but were not sure how much influence these had had. Another group reported having written to all the candidates standing in their local elections, together with other local councillors, inviting them to a meeting: only one reply had subsequently been received and this was a refusal. Hence, in this study, where service users tried to shape and form the basis for consultation, they lost direct access to established routes to the decision-making process.

Participants in this study also felt undermined in their involvement by the emphasis placed by professional staff on 'representativeness'. A number of service users believed that they could not attend external committees as a representative of their centre or service users more generally, because they did not think that they could be representative of that larger constituency. Integral to this concern was the fear that members of an external committee would level exactly this allegation against a user representative and the user would be able to do nothing except agree. Yet few steps were taken to address the question of representation. Some service users' representatives saw this problem as needing the opportunity to communicate clearly with those they were supposed to represent and in some of the centres studied, staff did give support to representatives, making sure they had time to prepare for meetings beforehand and debrief afterwards. More typically such efforts weren't made and user representatives felt isolated and confused about their role.

Another difficulty for these service users was adapting to the idea that they were now sitting on decision-making bodies on which professionals who might be, and in some cases were, responsible for making decisions about their individual treatment were also present. It had implications for the degree to which they felt able to be honest and one even talked about fear of 'reprisal'. At one day centre this was explained in a different way – 'well you are dependent on them [staff members] for those little favours – a lift here, advice there – that aren't really part of their job. You don't want to upset the goodwill'. The need to assist service users and professionals to make this transition, to put aside the effects of years of experience of inequality in the mental health system is a constant theme of the Canadian literature on user involvement strategies (Valentine and Capponi, 1989; Vandergang, 1996; Wilson, S., 1996; Lord *et al.*, 1998).

Fit for the purpose

Two other UK projects demonstrate the value of designing consultation strategies that attempt both to recognise the difficulties that service users may have in being able to express their voice, and to establish specific channels through which that voice is to be heard. The experience of these projects reflects users' uncertainty about the validity of their opinions after years of experiencing services and attitudes that have undermined their beliefs, and also their unfamiliarity with formal decision-making and planning forums. Pugh and Richards (1996) describe a consultation exercise involving 130 service users conducted in 1993 within the context of the All Wales Strategy for Mental Illness. The consultation took place in groups specifically set-up for the purpose, that were facilitated by service users who received some training for the task, and built on the experience of an earlier more limited exercise. Attention was paid to providing user-friendly environments and ease of access, including the provision of travel expenses for the participants. Subsequently professional workers and facilitators reported increased confidence among participants. This was particularly true of those who acted as members of patients councils and planning groups, who felt that the exercise gave them an opportunity to gauge the feelings of the 'constituency' they represented and feel that they had their support in putting views forward.

Pilgrim and Waldron (1998) report on a similar exercise in one NHS trust involving a small number of service users meeting a number of times. One important characteristic was that group members were not simply passively consulted but also had responsibility for negotiating subsequent changes. While the authors are clear that the group was not seen as a therapy group, they identify clear benefits for its members. Hence, many group members initially clung to bio-medical explanations of their experiences and were inclined to interpret their skill deficits and weaknesses as a function of their illness. Later members began to challenge this as an impediment to agency and challenged group members who used their illness as an explanation of unreliability. This transformation in attitude was matched by the development of skills in working in group settings and in negotiation.

A further problem identified in our own study (Bowl and Ross, 1994) was that agencies appeared to make no specific allowance for the exhausting and erratic experience of psychological distress which could mean that user representatives might not know until the last minute if they are able to attend a meeting. A number of users reported that when a user representative failed to attend an external meeting, no one made contact to find out why attendance had stopped. Indeed when the two user representatives on the joint care planning team in one authority stopped attending, apparently because of the stress that participation caused them, the reasons not only went unexplored but they were also not replaced.

This relative lack of interest in ensuring continuity of user representation and feedback indicates how important such participation is perceived as being to the decision-making process. The example also illustrates a potential disbenefit to particular individuals of involvement strategies, identified by users in this study. One important impact of psychological distress, and the disempowering experiences that often accompany it, can be the development of apathy and confusion. This may be accompanied by a consequent reluctance to engage with others and irregular attendance at centres. This means that it can be difficult for those users who want to become more active to achieve the support of their peers and share responsibility, so that some users who start out as enthusiastic and committed are soon burnt out by the relentless pressure of being always the spokesperson.

One particular user in the study, who was very active in terms of chairing internal discussions and sitting on various external committees, felt that the pressure of responsibility sat very heavily on him and contributed to the more frequent incidence of 'downers' he was experiencing. However, he believed that if he did not 'do these things', then nor would anyone else, so he battled on in the hope that someone else would soon be able to ease his burden. Interestingly, one of his fellow service users reported his own desire to get more involved in meetings and believed that as an articulate user, he had a valuable contribution to make in informing the professionals' perspective. He did not feel that he was going to be given the opportunity for greater participation, however, because of the greater experience of his colleague and the fact that he was not very well known among his peer group.

This was reflected in a particular paradox that occurred in several of the groups involved in the study – criticism over the lack of opportunities to get involved accompanied by a reluctance to participate more when such opportunities presented themselves.

Differences in perception between professionals and service users of the problems of continuity of user representation and 'burn-out' have been documented in Vandergang's survey of involvement strategies adopted by agencies in Toronto.

> While some agencies discussed continuity in neutral terms (for example, 'it's difficult for participants to sustain and follow up interest'), others used rather negative wording, referring to consumers/survivors' 'inability to commit' and 'lack of... accountability'. One agency stated that it's 'stressful for task-oriented agencies not to be able to count on people'. ...Interestingly, no-one conceived of the problem of continuity in terms of unrealistic or unfair expectations on the part of agencies. (Vandergang, 1996:159)

Other models of 'involvement' (broadly understood) also need to be considered here. As we have seen, mental health service users are increasingly being drawn into mainstream services as trainers, educators, researchers and policy workers. Such developments have a particular significance in recognising the contribution of 'user knowledge' to professional practice and policy development. These developments are often in their early stages and there is little research evidence to draw on which can help us understand what impact such involvement has on service users. However, one of the authors is currently working with a group of user trainers to help them evaluate their work, both in terms of the impact of the training they provide on its recipients, but also the impact of being involved in this way on themselves. Nine months into this project the user trainers reported improved confidence and feelings of self-worth, the development of specific skills, and support from within the group described as 'second to none', 'amazing', 'unique'. The particular significance of this experience of being supported and valued within the group was related to a capacity to build the trust which was often lacking in relationships experienced outside this context.

Overall, despite the tendency of many professionals to view consultation and participation strategies in terms of therapy, the evidence about their impact on individual service users is limited. Several studies, including our own, report benefits to service users of changed attitudes, increased confidence and the development of committee and group working skills.

Research in the area, however, is undeveloped and relatively unsystematic and is often conducted by enthusiasts for user involvement. There is little evidence of the impact on service users' experience of symptoms or use of services. What research does show, however, is that benefits are enhanced where the purpose of consultation is clear and special attention is paid to the conditions necessary to facilitate the contribution of service user representatives. Where this is not done the effects can be confusion, frustration and a reinforcement of feelings of disempowerment.

Self-help, autonomous action and benefits for service users

The concept and practice of self-help has a long history. The apolitical connotations of the concept mean that many contemporary user groups would not describe themselves in this way, although may find themselves so described by others and may acknowledge that self-help is a result if not the prime purpose of their actions (Barnes and Shardlow, 1997). The terms: pressure groups, consumer groups, advocacy groups and interest groups have all been used to describe autonomous groups comprising service users (see Barnes, 1999c), while their action has also been analysed by reference to theories of new social movements (Rogers and Pilgrim, 1991; Barnes, 1999c).

The key distinction we have drawn in our analysis is between separate organisation on the part of mental health service users and action from within service systems to invite or enable users to play some role in the decision making process (if only by providing feedback on existing services). Official action to involve users may result in autonomous groups taking part in deliberative forums with officials and, within this context, service users then become subject to the rules made by officials. But the separate existence of such groups also means they have at least some space to determine their own agendas and to proactively pursue their own objectives rather than always acting in responsive mode. This is different from the situation in which individuals are invited to take part in an official consultation exercise (or indeed to take part as participants in decision *taking* forums), but who do not have a user-controlled group or organisation as a point of reference and support. *A priori* we would suggest that autonomous action is more capable of enabling users to empower themselves than is the invitation to take part in a forum where the rules are made by officials.

Segal *et al.* (1993), for example, focus on the way user involvement within mental health service agencies is compromised by the 'paradox of empowerment', arguing that 'if empowerment... can be initiated and sustained only by those who seek power and self-determination, then it cannot legitimately be conferred by others who can define the parameters of such power' (ibid.: 708). They identify particular concerns over the way that the areas over which service users are 'allowed' to exercise power are determined by professionals, about the continuing power gradient between service users and professionals and about the background of coercion that underpins the work of such agencies. In contrast, self-help organisations are seen as seeking to empower in four ways:

1. by providing models that emphasise the achievements and potential of service users and hence counter stigma;
2. by giving individuals access to the resources and skills needed to reach their personal goals;
3. by giving service users control over and responsibility for organisation policy;
4. by collectively seeking changes in wider society.

Research exploring the impacts of self-help groups in a variety of health contexts have reported positive results relating to: improvements in mental state, improvements in knowledge, improvements in quality of life, increased chances of survival and reduced hospitalisation (research summarised at http://www.cmhc.com/selfhelp/research.htm).

Self-help organisations represent an important element of the consumer/survivor movement in Canada and the USA that has not yet reached the same prominence or level of development in the UK. Watkins and Callicutt (1997), indeed, report that there are 75,000 self-help groups (broadly defined and including relatives' groups) with 10–15 million members operating in the USA. Riessman and Carroll (1995) set the number somewhat lower, citing 7.5 million participants but they make a distinction between mutual aid groups and 'self-help writ large', which would also include professionally facilitated groups that we would see as outside our definition of autonomous action.

Self-help groups have also been successful in attracting official encouragement and financial support. For example, the Consumer/Survivor Development Initiative (CSDI) in Ontario attracts over 3.2 million dollars per annum. These organisations have many purposes – some, for example, focus exclusively on one particular aspect of the need to address the ability of those experiencing distress to survive and participate within the broader community. Hence some take the form of employment co-operatives – an analysis of the 36 organisations funded by the CSDI included six such co-operatives operating in catering, commercial cleaning and courier services (Trainor *et al.*, 1997). Other self-help organisations manage supported housing schemes.

Other organisations have a more generic focus, often worked out in detail as the organisation develops and its members establish its most appropriate functions. The examples of such organisations described by Trainor *et al.* (1997) show mutual support, cultural activities and advocacy to be the most common activities. The development of educational resources and skills training for other survivors, public education and education work with professionals are also important. Yet other such organisations either focus almost entirely on advocacy or appear closer in purpose to more conventional service agencies, taking on cases and providing relatively similar services but are distinguished from them by being managed by committees of service users and often by employing survivors themselves as front-line workers,.

This in itself indicates that there are differences in the philosophical orientations of self-help organisations that reflect the broad differences in outlook that we outline in Chapter 3. Nor do all who describe themselves as self-help organisations reflect identically the broad principles of the self-help movement outlined by Riessman and Carroll (1995). They are all fundamentally based upon the idea that difficulties can best be resolved by realising the potential strengths within a self-help unit (individual, group or community) rather than by external intervention controlled by experts. All place an accent on the importance of experienced-based wisdom and the notion that consumers can also be producers of help and services – what Toffler (1980) refers to as 'prosumers'. Importantly for the focus of this book, however, not all interpret the ideas of democracy in the private sphere and the importance of user involvement in the same way. Hence some have structures which reflect participative democratic ideals, while others employ workers and even managers with similar delegated powers to those that would be found in a conventional service agency.

There are also differences in the relative commitment of self-help organisations to internal and external goals. Riessman and Carroll (op. cit.), in countering claims that self-help diverts the energy of disadvantaged groups from necessary political activity, recognise that the initial activities of self-help organisations are likely to focus upon two complementary activities – mutual support for individual members and consciousness-raising. These will help develop skills and change in individuals but are also likely to lead to an awareness of restrictions on what can be achieved without external changes. This may well encourage the development of external activity to create change – collective self-advocacy. The earlier processes of developing shared perspectives and understanding and developing skills in groups should, in turn, have prepared the organisations for such external activity – indeed it has been suggested that in Canada, groups have been precipitated into external activity without developing this essential strength first – to the detriment of the effectiveness of the service user movement (Everett, 1998).

Segal *et al.* (1993) go further, arguing that the development of such advocacy is necessary if user-run organisations are to really be effective. Otherwise they will continue to have a secondary, responsive role – filling in gaps or covering the inadequacies of the state psychiatric system, dealing with the consequences of other aspects of society – providing complements or alternatives to a system that they are never able to change. Indeed they argue that it is impossible not to have some external influence, because the very existence of a self-help organisation run by, for example, survivors of psychiatric treatment for depression must influence public perceptions of the capabilities of those survivors – the existence of the organisation effectively redefines the implications of depression. Riessman and Carroll (op. cit.) support this idea, citing the particular example of Alcoholics Anonymous, who eschew all political activity. However, key members are often consulted on local and national issues and their activities have dramatically influenced views of both alcohol misuse and its treatment. Nonetheless it is clear that the balance of external and internal activity varies greatly across the spectrum of self-help organisations.

What is known about the effectiveness of self-help organisations? Well clearly they have been able to demonstrate to funders their ability to deliver certain valued and desired outcomes or funds would have been withdrawn. They also must strike some resonance with other service users/survivors as the movement proliferates and presses for more funding.

The 'helper-therapy principle'

Important at the theoretical level is the 'helper-therapy principle' (Riessman and Carroll, 1995) which stresses the benefits that accrue from reciprocity in the helping process. It is a particular paradox that those who most need help in a mental health context, because they suffer from disadvantage that is characterised by lack of self-esteem or self-worth and who experience stigma from that disadvantage, may be reluctant to seek help because it may reinforce those feelings. This is particularly true if help is perceived as taking place within a relationship characterised by a clear power gradient between an individual with little insight into their experience and a powerful, knowledgeable professional. This may simply reinforce ideas of dependency and incompetence. In contrast, within organisations practising mutual aid, an individual may be a helper one day, someone receiving help the next. Indeed giving and receiving help might well be part of the same transaction. Hence help-giving will be informed by the experience of receiving help and should be more sensitive to that experience and help received within a more equal relationship. More fundamentally, members when giving help, will experience the benefits of a sense of competence and self-esteem and the social recognition that this valued role brings. It may also help them by bringing a new perspective on their own similar experiences.

Typically members of self-help groups report that their membership and the responsibility that they have the chance to exercise is empowering. Individuals report the development of organisational and vocational skills and a growth in self-esteem, self-confidence and well-being that accompanies the recognition of their experiential knowledge and the opportunity to act as role models for other service users. Trainor *et al.*'s (1997) study of 653 members of self-help organisations, who they identify as having experienced serious mental health problems, reported a feeling of having more choices, being more in control and having an enhanced ability to cope day to day. Much of the latter development was attributed to respondents' growth in knowledge about possibilities and restrictions imposed by their distress that developed from sharing awareness with others. Far from providing simply a sheltered 'ghetto' experience, 60 per cent of respondents also reported increased contacts with non-survivors arising from their enhanced feelings of self-respect and that they had enhanced their interpersonal skills.

Barnes and Shardlow (1997) place a different emphasis in their analysis of three UK user groups, reflecting on benefits in terms of the very needs service users themselves identify as central. They allow members, through their activities in the groups to reintegrate, to participate in society in ways which we expect to derive from our unwritten notion of citizenship. Hence they are able to reclaim some of what is lost through the exclusion often deriving from mental distress. User groups help service users to realise the potential of their legal and procedural rights, offering information and support in claiming benefits, and in using complaints and appeals procedures. Through their activities in raising public awareness they help counter the effects of stigma and discrimination. They facilitate participation in leisure, education and training (of both themselves and others) and they may even help to counter the most significant structural factors, for example, by facilitating employment.

Importantly such action opens up possibilities to move beyond the identity of 'service user':

> In some ways it turned out to be a positive step for me. It changed my life around from something that was killing me, virtually, to something that I finally got some kind of reward in.

> it's given me a life and without it I wouldn't have dreamed of doing half the things I do now. It's given me confidence, assurance... I get up now and speak at a conference quite happily. A few years ago I would have no more done that than fly!

> there's quite a few that have come here and when they came they wouldn't say boo to a goose. They've been here a bit, you can't shut them up – which is what we want to hear! (Mental health user activists quoted in Barnes and Shardlow, 1996)

This is not to say that user-run organisations are always themselves perfectly empowering. Particularly where self-help organisations receive funding from government institutions, there may be conflicts between attempting to facilitate maximum user involvement and control and meeting the service level targets set by funding bodies. Conflicts may also arise, for workers employed on conventional employment contracts by self-help organisations, between encouraging user involvement and meeting the organisations' expectations of their management skills. Similarly it is easy for advocacy organisations, in their desire to meet external demands for advice and training or to carry influence, to rely on a few individuals with experience to drive the organisation at the expense of internal opportunities for other service users to develop skills, experience and confidence.

Athena McLean's study of the 'Quad', a consumer-run community resource centre in the USA, highlights some of the problems (McLean,

1995). She found little sense of empowerment among the centre's users or confidence that they could alter decisions made there that impacted directly upon them. This in turn she traced to senior staff (themselves service users) pathologising members in terms of their diagnostic labels, separating themselves from a responsibility for dirty, menial work in the centre, unreasonably exploiting volunteers' preparedness to support the centre's work and in other ways adopting autocratic control. While some of this could be traced to issues of personal style, much resulted from the need to maintain external relationships with funders and those the organisation wished to influence. A crisis developed and eventually the organisation had to change personnel and reappraise its mission. McLean suggests that this is not an unusual experience within USA self-help organisations many of which, she suggests, suffer from 'social amnesia about their mission':

> Unless consumers who are invested in the politically empowering mission of the psychiatric consumer movement succeed in sharing their vision with newcomers to the movement, it is likely that consumer-run alternatives will continue to move in directions that fall severely short of their espoused goals, become little more than extensions of the traditional mental health sector and appeal to funders more than their users. Should this continue the unique potential of self-help to promote recovery in ways that depart in concept and form from traditional mental health services will simply not be realised. (ibid.: 1067)

Nonetheless self-help organisations have been shown to reach the sorts of targets set within clinical discourse as indications of recovery. Gordon *et al.* (1982), for example, compared the experience of discharged patients allocated randomly to a conventional after-care programme or to the programme plus referral to a mutual aid group. Only half as many of the group referred for mutual aid required hospitalisation in the subsequent study period (17.5 per cent as opposed to 35 per cent), their stays in hospital were shorter and twice as many functioned in the community without any further contact with the formal mental health services. Kurtz and Chambon (1987) report similar reductions in rates of hospitalisation and shorter stays. Trainor *et al.*'s (1997) study shows significant reductions in contacts with crisis services, outpatient visits and most dramatically in inpatient days. Comparing the year after initial membership with a year before they show a drop from a mean of 48 inpatient days to 4!

Joint working

Overall the evidence suggests positive outcomes for individuals from user self-run organisations but that this can be compromised where relationships with conventional providers and founders become too restrictive or the adoption of the practices of conventional service agencies cause them to lose sight of their founding principles. There are indeed those who see absolute separation from conventional services as necessary if the essential energy and oppositional nature of the users/survivors movement is to be sustained. Involvement in consultation exercises and in service contracts is seen as a distraction and bringing the danger of incorporation (Forbes and Sashidharan, 1997).

Could a third way – joint working – offer different benefits? Could initiatives where service users worked in genuine partnership with professionals and administrators compromise the deep structures that maintain professional power even when users are invited into consultation exercises within service organisations while also facilitating genuine user influence? Is there indeed any evidence of such joint working and what is its effect? We have struggled to find such examples in the UK – rather being faced by participative exercises firmly reflecting the needs of service organisations and independent organisations struggling to exercise influence in their relationships with media, politicians and administrators without being too compromised.

Perhaps the clearest examples of such joint working come from the coalitions and partnerships between service users and allies such as professional organisations and family groups that have formed in both Canada and the USA, often for a relatively short-term and often targeted around specific one-off changes in policy (Church and Reville, 1989; Wilson, S., 1996). Nelson (1994) provides a useful account of the coalition formed to advocate for housing and community support programmes in Waterloo (Ontario) and reflects upon similar campaigns in Vermont and Maryland among others. However, while he reports on their achievements in creating policy and resource changes (discussed in more depth in Chapter 6) there is little here about their impact on the service users involved of working for change in such a context.

Such coalitions are starting to develop in the UK (for example, around research and policy organisations – as discussed in Chapter 3). These new types of relationship between professionals and users demonstrate a greater equality at the interpersonal level, although such relationships still operate in conditions where power over resources is very unequally distributed and where the options open to professional researchers, educators and policy analysts mean that they could redirect their interests and energies elsewhere if the experience fails to deliver.

Changing the professionals and the public

The impact of the movement as a whole on professional administrators and practitioners can be seen in the acknowledgement of the need to take a different view of service users' capability. Sinnika McCabe is director of the Bureau of Community Mental Health in Wisconsin and writes:

> Increasingly, the service recipient is being viewed as an equal partner in the treatment process, not a passive service user. Mature mental health systems recognise that there is virtually no difference in intelligence, ability, and talents between people who have experienced treatment in the mental health system and those who have not. The difference is in perspective, and this different point of view is viewed as valuable, worthwhile and important. (McCabe and Unzicker, 1995: 61)

While this may be an optimistic view of the extent to which service users' perspectives are yet accepted as an essential alternative view, it has also to an extent been recognised in the UK. Hence, there has been a succession of pieces of legislation, just as there was in the USA from the mid-1980s onwards, which continue to emphasise the importance of involving service users in planning, managing, evaluating and delivering services. This is stressed in the NHS and Community Care Act, in *Building Bridges* (DoH, 1995) and in the new partnership initiatives discussed in Chapter 3. Of course it can be argued that some of the impetus came from arguments within the academy but can it really be said that they were in turn developed independently of the existence and growing strength of the movement itself?

There is also emphasis on the importance of users' perspectives impacting upon the training of professionals in the UK. Ramon and Sayce (1993) and Curran (1997), for example, advocate strongly for their reflection in the training of social workers and Hopton (1995) makes a case for changing community psychiatric nurse training in the same way. The 1994 mental health nursing review, *Working in Partnership*, further stressed the need for nurses to establish more egalitarian relationships with service users, involve them in planning and evaluation and respond more to service users' wishes and aspirations (DoH, 1994). The need to understand users' perspectives has also attained an important focus within Diploma in Social Work initial social work qualifying courses and the Central Council for Education and Training in Social Work's (CCETSW) Mental Health Social Work Award (post-qualifying training for those wishing to become Approved Social Workers). Indeed one of the criteria for acceptance on an Approved Social Worker programme is familiarity with and respect for collective users' perspectives. On both programmes it is necessary to specifically demonstrate competence in facilitating the service users' voice.

It is also apparent that within the UK, much as has been noted in the USA (Segal *et al.*, 1993; Riessman and Carroll, 1995), service user organisations are recognised as 'experts' in their field and as such are drawn into consultations on practice and policy developments even where it is not a statutory requirement. Just as 'The Wisconsin Bureau of Community Mental Health biennial work plan for 1993–95 states that no work groups or task forces may be established without including consumer/survivors on them' (McCabe and Unzicker, 1995: 67), a number of key UK organisations like CCETSW are thus inclined to include service user consultation in a wide range of policy deliberations.

The apparent acceptance by professional administrators and practitioners of the need for greater user involvement needs to be viewed carefully, however. First, as we argued in Chapter 3, enthusiasm might well be greater among policy makers than practitioners – not least because user perspectives may sometimes be seen as offering help in their own battles to impose change on reluctant professionals. Also service user desire for more control over what happens to them can be interpreted as supporting reductions in services delivered by professionals and their replacement by more, perhaps less well resourced, consumer-run alternatives. This has different implications from a desire for professional services that are more responsive to service users' preferences, which might well be more expensive (see for example Everett, 1998). It is also important to reflect back on our earlier assertion that one reason for the apparent consensus around the desirability of service user involvement is that different meanings are attached to the concept. In particular therapists tend to focus largely on its therapeutic benefits. Hence apparent acceptance may actually result from differences in understanding of what is meant by user involvement.

This can be illustrated by a personal salutary experience encountered during our own field work. Having met the staff at one particular mental health day centre, we were impressed by their enthusiasm and endorsement of user involvement strategies and were invited to the next users' committee. This turned out to be a committee where the roles of chair and secretary were both in the hands of staff 'facilitators', who also decided the bulk of the agenda. The meeting was long and included very little participation by service users other than to provide answers to direct questions from the staff members. Afterwards we stayed to talk to the service user members on their own and were treated to an even longer but considerably more active meeting. It was led by the service users and featured sophisticated critiques of the way the centre was run; of the limited functioning of the committee and how their views were taken seriously when they were useful to staff in pursuing their particular agenda, such as when they were fighting to protect jobs at the centre, but otherwise ignored; and of the limitations and strengths of local services generally. Later, staff members expressed satisfaction with the committee's functioning, which they saw as giving service users as much of a say as they could handle.

Church's study of the consultation process in Ontario over possible legislative changes needed to underpin the community-based mental health system recommended by the Graham Report, is also instructive. While the administrators involved insisted that their views of the central needs of service users and their ability to articulate these had been positively altered by the process, they also expressed shock and discomfort with how service users expressed their views and with the level of emotional exchange that user consultation drew them into. It seems that consultation was all right in principle, particularly if it remained within the strictly controlled conventional committee format laid down for the exercise, but the reality proved more painful than had been anticipated for commission members and some were clearly reluctant to engage with service users in the same way again (Church, 1996).

Baker (1997) is one advocate of the potential of partnerships between professionals and service users in planning, evaluating and delivering services to constructively transform the views held of each other but to what extent professional attitudes have yet been transformed by the movement is open to question. There is little solid research evidence to inform us, although we examine interesting material on staff resistance to greater user influence in Chapter 6. Kent and Read (1998) also identify largely positive views of the likely benefits of employment of service users within mental health services and of their involvement in planning among a range of mental health professionals in New Zealand. To what extent these attitudes would really be evidenced in practice is not clear, however, as the authors note that development of user involvement strategies is at an early stage. They also identify that professionals with a greater commitment to the medical model were less likely to know about user involvement in their organisations and were more likely to see negative consequences arising from it.

Hence we are left to strike a balance between the evidence of increased policy and training commitments to greater user involvement with little detailed evidence of real attitude change among professionals, some evidence of confusion about and in some cases resistance to the reality of such involvement and continuing perceptions on the part of service users of too little change. It is also true that professional attitudes are shaped in a similar context to those that influence public views. Again there is too little concrete evidence of how these might have been changed by a mental health service users movement demonstrating a greater potential for agency among service users than might previously been assumed. On the one hand we see public acquiescence to the changes that have encouraged greater user involvement but to what extent are the skills so developed recognised outside the mental health field? (Everett, 1998). Such a recognition would be a clear signal of a real change. Instead the media report continuing resistance to the location of residential establishments and supported housing for former psychiatric patients within local communities. We also see apparent popular support for proposals to significantly restrict the liberties of those experiencing distress that seem in open contradiction to the idea that service users are capable of exercising greater autonomy over their lives and the services that so dramatically affect them.

6

Changing the system

Within Chapter 5 we set out to examine evidence of the impact of user self-organisation and involvement in the planning and delivery of services on both service users themselves and the attitudes of individuals. In contrast, this chapter looks for evidence of influence on the structures and policies of the organisations that deliver mental health services. We described towards the end of Chapter 5 how, since the late 1980s, both legislation and policy guidance impacting upon mental health services have stressed the need for service user involvement in the planning and delivery of services. We also described how, even where legislation does not specifically require it, user involvement has become established as good practice. In themselves these developments would appear to indicate changes in the ideas of those managing and providing services and perhaps in the minds of the public who provide policy makers with a democratic mandate to make changes on their behalf. Nonetheless, we also alluded to the fears that both in Canada (Everett, 1998) and the USA (McLean, 1995) strategies encouraging increased user involvement had not necessarily produced real changes in mainstream mental health provision. Indeed, diverting the energy of the movement away from its oppositional role may have lessened the momentum for change it had generated.

In an earlier summary of ideas about the evolution of social movements, Everett describes how as a movement begins to take effect it passes through the stage of institutionalisation – '[the point at which] the government (usually the target of protest) has been forced to develop a number of coping strategies in order to deal with the movement; some may entail its eradication, others may involve its incorporation' (Everett, 1994: 56). Perhaps the victories gained in legislating for users' voices to be heard should be seen as part of a coping strategy designed to lessen rather than accentuate the impact of the movement – clearly the view of some UK commentators (Forbes and Sashidharan, 1997). Certainly Everett's analysis of how mental health services absorbed the impact of three earlier movements – the asylum, mental hygiene and deinstitution-alisation movements – without undergoing fundamental changes is a chilling warning (Everett, 1994).

Nonetheless, much of what has been written about the UK to date remains speculative and research clearly delineating the success or other-wise of service user interventions is difficult to find. To some extent this reflects the domination of the experimental approach within the medical research paradigm and the reluctance of those funding research to support other approaches. Yet the real world is not a laboratory, experimental control on the many variables that may influence the nature of mental health service provision is rarely achievable and the experimental approach seldom appropriate. Hence our attempt in this chapter to piece together the evidence of service organisations responding to the perspec-tives offered by service users is drawn from a variety of sources. These include our own experience, the published work of others and conversa-tions with movement activists.

Surveys, focus groups and consultation exercises

Service organisations striving for service user input into planning and decision-making have used a variety of methods including feedback from surveys and other forms of research. In this case the views of service users are systematically sought but the results are interpreted by others without service users being involved in their application or participating directly in the forums in which they are considered. Nonetheless, propo-nents of this approach in the UK are often enthusiastic about its effects. Bailey (1997), for example, describes a Family Health Services Authority consultation exercise which looked at the delivery of primary mental health care and involved ten self-selected service users. The service users voiced well-established views about GPs' poor understanding of mental health, their failure to really listen to service users and their failure to explain the consequences of treatment fully. They also appear to have endorsed the benefits of surgery-based counselling and a GP-held register of patients with mental health problems. Bailey reports that, following this consultation, GPs have been supplied with information leaflets for users and carers and some have received special funding to enable the employment of extra staff, including counsellors, to develop mental health work. Service users are also to be involved in training for primary care staff on mental health issues. These are significant developments and, while details of the wider context and other possible influences on them are not reported, to a degree they clearly have to be seen as influenced by the service user input.

Hannigan *et al.* (1997) report on a larger consultation with five focus groups of service users in three London boroughs. This sought to establish service users' views on what they assumed mental health and social functioning to be and what they thought would help achieve them. These are key targets for improvement within UK government health policies (DoH, 1992). Ultimately the consultation produced answers that would be familiar to those involved in the users/survivors movement. Social functioning was seen in terms of having relationships with friends and intimates, being integrated into normal life, having sufficient money and not having to deal with stigma. Mental health was perceived in terms of self-esteem, coping and self-determination and the implications for services covered the need for refuge, counselling, consistent support and genuine relationships with service providers. While clearly the exercise created some impact among the researchers (employees of local health trusts) there is no evidence given of any direct service changes. This should not surprise us. In an interesting analysis of some of the conceptual and practical difficulties of 'consumer satisfaction' surveys, Stallard (1996) points out how commonly researchers fail to specify any service changes arising from their studies. Some specifically report receiving no indications for change and those that do appear to involve identifiable changes in mainstream mental health services – a study by Jones and Lodge (1991) reporting improvements in an outpatient waiting area and that by Bond *et al.* (1992) improvements to the inpatient service at one Shropshire hospital – hardly represent significant moves forward for the agenda of the users/survivors movement.

In contrast, the user consultation exercise described by Pugh and Richards (1996) involved a large number of service users in a more interactive and participative exercise facilitated by their peers. The themes emerging from this exercise were very much in line with the central concerns of the users/survivors movement – the need for users to receive more information on treatment and share the decision as to whether to accept it or not; the need for 24-hour access to help and greater availability of talking therapies; the damaging impact of dismissive professional attitudes and the benefits of advocacy services; and the central importance of extended housing and work options among them. Pugh and Richards report that subsequently the record of the consultation has begun to influence service planning and provision. They attribute to it a number of changes, including the piloting of a non-medical respite facility and a 24-hour helpline and the establishment of a professional advocacy service in one hospital. There is, however, no reflection on the role of other potential influences on these changes such as, for example, the impetus given to service development by the All Wales Strategy, of which the exercise was a small part.

Similarly Carpenter and Sbaraini (1996) report how interviews with individual service users and a subsequent consultation exercise involving service users were important to the construction of local Care Programme Approach procedures designed to enhance the effectiveness of user input into individual care planning. A number of service users were subsequently surveyed to assess the efficacy of these procedures and identified continuing problems in gaining adequate information about the effects of medication and alternatives to it and about complaints procedures. Dissatisfaction with some element of their care was reported by 79 per cent. There is no report of further developments that might have addressed these outstanding concerns.

Following through

A potentially more empowering form of user involvement involves service users more actively in following through directly the service implications of their ideas. This was an element built into the exercise in one health trust reported by Pilgrim and Waldron (1998). This involved a group of a dozen service users, initially facilitated by two professional workers. They met frequently over a sustained period, identifying a number of issues they wished to pursue, including the need for 24-hour services, more access to advocacy and improved communication and information from professionals. In its first year the group successfully negotiated Sunday opening for a day centre using the evidence provided by a survey of carers that they had conducted; initiated discussions which led to the health authority appointing a paid specialist advocate at the local mental health inpatient unit; and assembled and published a user information booklet with financial assistance from the local health authority.

A different sort of forum, on which service users were joined by carers, local authority staff and voluntary sector personnel is described by Milewa (1997). One health authority and social services area established a series of regular forums that would report recommendations, decisions and requests to the local joint care planning team for mental health. After two years the impact of the forums was reviewed. Only 11 (less than 20 per cent) of the interventions by the forums are described as 'successes' and over half drew no response at all. There were few successes on the critical issues like funding priorities, which were of greatest concern to the forums. Indeed successes predominantly involved the forums' own organisation or that of other aspects of the planning process.

It is more difficult to estimate the impact of the regular involvement of service users in mainstream planning and management committees, not least because of the difficulties of linking changes to the contributions of those individual members. We have discussed, however, the limited achievements that individuals in our own study (Bowl and Ross, 1994) identified within formal planning systems and on user committees and Lindow (1994) is among those critical of the impact of user participation in patient councils.

Achievements in partnership

Involvement of the UK users/survivors movement in working together with other organisations is as yet a relatively rare phenomenon. It has happened for short-term local campaigns but coalitions and partnerships are a less common feature of the UK mental health scene than appears to be the case in the USA and Canada. Perhaps they are features of a more mature users' movement, where a greater strength and internal coherence has been established that makes it easier to make the sort of compromises necessary to working together.

While, as we argued earlier, experimental designs are seldom appropriate, research in this area reveals some of the benefits that can accrue from a thoughtfully constructed, systematic approach. One analysis, based on resource mobilisation theory (Jenkins 1983, 1987) carefully assesses the impact of a coalition of survivors, professionals, relatives and other community organisations in its attempts to increase the supply of supported housing and aftercare services sensitive to survivor preferences in the Waterloo region of Ontario (Nelson, 1994). The coalition was successful in achieving a major expansion in the number of supported housing spaces and more funding for community health programmes in the region (at a greater rate of growth than of health expenditure generally or of mental health expenditure in the province as a whole). The role of specific activities in achieving this success and the

particular role played by the 15 per cent of members of the coalition identified as survivors is not clear, however. Also other influences are identified – important local and provincial political changes and an
organisational infrastructure, through which to implement changes relatively easily, are identified as important to this success.

Both Church and Reville (1989) and Nelson (1994) identify other
coalition achievements in Toronto, in transforming the supply of
supported housing, and in Vermont and Maryland in shifting resources to
the community rather than institutions. All were characterised by the
achievement of broad consensus within the coalition, favourable local
political control, and well-established organisational support for the
coalition. In contrast, less successful coalitions reported by Nelson in
Manitoba, Long Beach and Connecticut were hampered by resistance
from the ruling political administration and a resistant bureaucracy.

Partnership is not, however, completely absent from the UK scene.
The separation of service purchasing from provision in health services
in the early 1990s in the UK resulted in opportunities for users to take
part in decision making about what services should be provided and
what the contract specifications for such services should be. Thus, in
Nottingham, Nottingham Advocacy Group (NAG) became involved in
what was known as 'PUG' – the Purchasing for Users Group – making
detailed inputs particularly to the specification of requirements to
provide information about services and medication and to provide aftercare services following discharge. Their close working relationships
with the statutory services also led to them being called in to look at
what was going wrong in a day centre which had experienced a sharp
drop in the numbers using it. The outcome was a major reorganisation of
the centre's management that drew services users in directly (information from private correspondence). In Newcastle the Mental Health
Services Consumer Group has similarly had a significant role in relation
to the purchasing or commissioning of mental health services. Harrison
(1993) highlights their role in the establishment of a review of the
district health authority's continuing central emphasis on centralised
hospital-based services and in influencing quality standards for
rehabilitation and continuing care. She also identifies how their involvement in planning and contract specification have also led to other opportunities for users to shape services. For example, they have been invited
to help a local community mental health team develop greater consumer
involvement in the services it provides.

Advantages of independence

Many service users remain ambivalent about the advantages of either participative or partnership strategies. In particular, based on their own experience, many doubt professionals' ability or willingness to use their power to further service users' interests rather than their own (Williams and Lindley, 1996). Hence they prefer to organise separately and attempt to engage with and change services and other features of society that influence their lives from outside the formal mechanisms of the system.

There are many forms that such autonomous action can take. In our study of three local authorities (Bowl and Ross, 1994) a user group had formed at one centre which had once suffered from a poor public perception due to its history as a place of containment. Over the previous few years, a more energetic and 'enlightened' staff group had encouraged a therapeutic and enabling environment. When a new manager took over and wanted to return to a more disciplined and essentially disempowering regime, the users, with support from some staff members, wrote to their local Social Services Department expressing their dissatisfaction and demanding an enquiry. The manager was subsequently relocated and the centre returned to its more facilitative path. Even though users understood that an enquiry might mean that Social Services Department staff would 'interrogate' them and make them feel uncomfortable and afraid, users reported that they had been fighting for *their* service and were prepared to face the possible intimidation. The experience contributed to building confidence in these service users to feel they could effect change.

Other independent centre-based groups or broader forums in the study were still relatively undeveloped although one local forum believed that it had been successful in changing professionals' attitudes towards users and that it had been this change which had enabled partnerships to become a reality. This forum believed that professionals do take their views seriously and new committees will often approach the forum to ask it to field a representative. Another relatively new forum had already organised a local conference on mental health issues and, through their efforts, a commitment to user involvement had been incorporated into their authority's joint strategy document.

Another important way in which the independent operation of service users' organisations can create change in statutory services is by providing alternative models of service. Examples of this are not as well established in the UK as the examples in the USA and Canada to which we have referred in Chapter 5. However, there can be little doubt of the influence, for example, of NAG's development of patient advocacy. This has now become recognised good practice and health authorities across the country have been keen to fund independent organisations to provide such a service or to directly employ someone providing an adapted version of it. Similarly many of the recommendations identified in guidance on work with women developed by the independent organisation Good Practices in Mental Health (Perkins *et al.*, 1996), which was informed by a significant service user input, have been integrated into mainstream services. There were, of course, other influences on this work, particularly from professionals, and it is not easy to locate the users/survivors movement's unique contribution. This, however, is not just a problem of analysis – it reflects the dynamics of how change occurs. Similarly, we would argue that the users/survivors movement has also contributed to the availability in GPs' surgeries of alternative treatments for psychological distress. It may be that professionals, disaffected with a strictly medical approach, have pursued these alternatives but this has certainly been given more legitimacy by the congruence of their ideas with articulated service users' preferences.

Resistance and representation

'While none claimed that the influence of user groups has resulted in a fundamental shift in the balance of power within the mental health system, it has provided a challenge to the prevailing system and has forced those in existing positions of power to look at things in different ways' (Barnes and Shardlow, 1997). If we were to try and summarise the overall impact of the users/survivors movement in the UK, it would be difficult to improve on this excerpt from one of our earlier observations. We might also add that developments are very patchy across the UK and even within individual health and social services authorities. In examining explanations for this pattern of uneven development, we look both at 'micro' level explanations – at what is happening in individual authorities and establishments – and at 'macro' level explanations – concerning what is happening at a national and, to a degree, international level.

First, despite the changes that have taken place, there is still considerable resistance on the part of some organisations and individuals to the encouragement of user involvement. This resistance takes many forms. Some involve overt incredulity about the capacity of users to exercise the levels of responsibility entailed. For example, while our own survey of principal officers responsible for mental health services indicated some commitment to user involvement, it also exposed the limits that can be placed upon it by perceptions of what services users can contribute (Bowl, 1996b). David Brandon argues that,

> the real sign of whether users have a say in running services lies in who appoints staff. There are five ways (in which this can happen):
>
> 1. No user involvement in staff appointments at all   VERY POOR
> 2. Users see people on the short list for coffee   POOR
> 3. One token user on appointments committee   FAIR
> 4. Half users/half staff on appointments committee   GOOD
> 5. Users make staff appointments with some staff help   EXCELLENT
>
> (Brandon, 1992: 11)

In the majority of authorities in our survey, service users had no involvement in staff selection and respondents were clear that in some cases there would be resistance to changing this:

> We have talked about it but it is too difficult to implement.

> They'd like to be but I don't think it is going to happen.

> It would be regarded as heresy.

> The fear is that, if users select, they will choose people who are useless – and there is no point if it is mere tokenism.

Indeed in only six (of 31) authorities was there formal representation of service users on selection panels and this was not always seen as unproblematic: 'users sometimes ask inappropriate questions', 'their view of who they want may conflict with everyone else – it's a difficulty'. There was irony too in two authorities offering equal opportunities policies as the reason why the representation was not possible within selection processes of one group who experience a particular lack of opportunity – service users!

One implication here seems to be that if service users behave differently or make different choices to the professionals this is a problem – yet surely the purpose of their involvement is to offer a different perspective! Of course involving service users may result in different decisions being made in this as well as other areas of activity. That is something that must be accepted if service user involvement is to be made a reality. Thought also needs to be given to how the form of existing forums might need to change to really facilitate that involvement – for example, are existing interview-based selection procedures necessarily the only way in which staff selection decisions must be made? Even in the authority in our study where service users were most clearly represented at all levels within the department, the respondent felt 'that this needs redesigning. We're fitting them into our structure at present. The whole thing needs further review'. Another remarked 'The department has no idea how to involve users, because if this is to be done then the language and structure of meetings has to be changed. If users are to become involved in a meaningful way, then the basic manner in which the organisation operates has to be changed, though training is an important element'.

The reference to training is important, particularly where service users are to be integrated into fixed structures and procedures. Why does it appear to be assumed that service users can develop the skills required in selection, planning and management forums without the training and support given to staff undertaking these tasks? In the authority in our study where user representation on selection panels was described as their most substantial achievement in user involvement, the establishment of training in selection and equal opportunities was seen as central to having made this possible.

There are other less overt forms of resistance. Perhaps the most frequently occurring is to doubt the 'representativeness' of service user nominees. One centre manager in our study, for example, had taken a deliberate decision not to have a user committee, since she believes that they are rarely 'representative' and 'give a platform to the loudest voices who don't necessarily reflect the views of the larger constituency'. There are many facets to this form of resistance – perhaps the most pernicious is to doubt the authenticity of the contribution of the articulate. 'The double bind that this places the consumer/survivor in is obvious: if you get well, you are really not representative; if you remain sick, you are too sick to be of any significant use or importance!' (McCabe and Unzicker, 1995: 64).

This is not to deny that there are very real problems around representation – for example: individuals being selected by staff rather than by their peers and particular service users being overwhelmed by the number of demands being placed upon them. Some of our respondents also had doubts as to the extent of direct service user involvement as opposed to that of carers and/or voluntary organisations in their consultation and participation processes. The limited numbers of user representatives involved also implies assumptions that a small number of service users can represent the diversity that exists among them. When this limited representation brought criticisms from service user groups or exposed fundamental differences in philosophy between different participants, this sometimes crystallised resistance to user involvement, which was seen as 'unsuccessful', and the user movement, which was 'riven by splits'.

None of these issues of appropriate representation, however, should be used as an excuse to prevent extensions of service user involvement, as it is only through the proliferation of these opportunities, that it will be possible to confront the issue of representation. Unfortunately, in our study, arguments about the representativeness of service users were regularly rehearsed by staff. Furthermore, it seemed that the constant articulation of the problem had been internalised by users and inhibited their enthusiasm for participation (Bowl, 1996a).

Conflicting demands, contrasting discourses

It would be wrong to 'blame' professionals for resisting increased service user involvement without attempting to understand it. Wadsworth and Epstein (1998) studied the development of a long-term dialogue between staff and service users at one psychiatric hospital. At first staff were very defensive and were keen to impress upon the investigators their own view that they feel disempowered themselves and felt a need for their own voice to be heard in the organisations in which they worked.

> However, the things of which staff most wanted to speak (emotional responses of fear, anxiety, rage, frustration and feelings of being badly treated) appeared to be simultaneously the things they felt most forbidden to say (and most forbade themselves saying) for fear of dismantling the carefully constructed 'difference' and 'othering' on which is based their authority and legalised powers as mental health professionals, as well as their own professional understanding of what they should do to 'provide care'. (Wadsworth and Epstein, 1998: 359)

There are several issues at stake here. First, a feature of health and social care organisations in recent history has been a tendency for management structures to attempt to exercise greater control over and surveillance of the activities of front-line professionals than previously. This has been attempted through the introduction of ideas borrowed from the private sector, such as systems of appraisal, job evaluation and case-load measurement. In these circumstances it is perhaps not difficult to see how many would be reluctant to concede to service users the control and authority that they perceive themselves as retaining. Our response would be that it is not a question of simply conceding authority. Developing user influence over policies and working practices can produce more appropriate provision and a therefore a greater shared sense of control over the problems with which both professionals and service users work. However, we can also see that this would involve a leap of faith that may not be easy for professionals feeling themselves to be under pressure.

More fundamentally within a mental health context, the dominant discourse in which professionals and service users are located, sees professionals as healthy, competent and rational and they are required to provide answers rather than questions, to know what is best. After all the scientific model, in restricting their focus of intervention, equips them with the information to be able to operate with a certain degree of certainty and offer the explanations for their experience that service users seek. In contrast, service users are sick, non-rational and dependent. In this context there is little room for staff uncertainty or to learn new ideas, accept alternative ways of seeing things posited by service users. The issue of the validity of emotional as opposed to intellectual knowledge is also relevant here. Seidler (1994) highlights how since the Enlightenment our culture has put explicit value on knowledge gathered and validated by the scientific method and has devalued emotional experience as a source of knowledge. The value base and training of mental health professionals reflect both the value of scientific knowledge and the importance of remaining emotionally detached (and unengaged emotionally with the service user) in order to be able to apply that scientific knowledge objectively. Such an approach is in direct opposition to what service users often want to convey. Perhaps, in this context, rather than be surprised by the inability of professionals to 'hear' the service users' voice, we should instead rejoice when we find examples of genuine dialogue. Certainly it is easy to see how, in the light of these fundamental differences, Wadsworth and Epstein found early attempts at dialogue gave rise to a 'closed loop cycle of claim/blame-defense-and-counter-claim/blame-defense' (op. cit.: 353).

Of course not all staff buy into the dominant discourse to the same degree and various professionals may see their value base differently. This indeed may be a problem in itself, if it leads to a failure to see the critical differences in perspective that must arise from the different roles performed by service users and professionals in the system. Many staff in the Wadsworth and Epstein study found it difficult to accept that they did not listen to service users and indeed take note and represent their views. A similar reluctance has been identified in a study of UK social workers. Many of these workers saw themselves as having a commitment working in partnership with service users while their practice showed little evidence of any such sharing (Marsh and Fisher, 1992). This perception on the part of professionals that they are able to take on service users' views and be their advocates may show a clear misunderstanding of what advocacy entails but it is not uncommon. Recently, in the capacity of external monitor, a long-term service user with whom we work, attended a series of training sessions on a programme of preparation for those seeking to become Approved Social Workers. The ASW role is seen by many as an essential socially informed balance to the medical view in decisions about whether or not service users are to be compulsorily detained (Gostin *et al.*, 1983; Barnes *et al.*, 1990). Nonetheless, it is the ASW who ultimately makes the application for detention based on the balance of those judgements. To his horror our colleague heard these professionals describing themselves as the 'service users' advocate' in the ASW assessment. Hopton (1995) also identifies how psychiatric nurses often identify themselves as sharing the service users' perspective in a struggle against dominance by psychiatry!

Staff in our own study also identified another related issue – that they were being asked to buy into two conflicting philosophies. One was about power and control and the other about involving service users and yet they were not being given the opportunity to work through the stresses to which this gives rise (Bowl, 1996a). The failure of many user involvement initiatives to confront this fundamental contradiction should not surprise us because it reflects an important tension that exists within the mental health system. The services and legislation that are in place are to an extent motivated by a concern and a desire to help but also by a societal fear and desire to control. While the former is admissible and reflected prominently in both national and local policy statements, the latter is often not on the open agenda. Indeed Wadsworth and Epstein highlight how the language used by professionals serves to conceal notions of fear and control – 'What might be for some staff "safe seclusion, necessary medication, a successful treatment option in x per cent of cases, unavoidable duty of care and behavioural modification" can be for many consumers "being locked up, forcibly injected, electrically shocked until you lost your memory, being assaulted, and treated like an animal"' (op. cit.: 374).

Yet concerns about control and the need to reassure a concerned public may always be underpinning political and managerial decisions and the professional practice that shapes the terrain in which user involvement takes place, restricting the potential for genuine user empowerment.

Different expectations and limited structures

The limited achievements of strategies encouraging involvement also reflect the different understandings of empowerment by different actors and the consequent goals they set for it: 'What is most frequently observed is the tendency to reduce the notion of empowerment to an individual attribute – to confound empowerment with personal competency, sense of control, or sense of self-efficacy – and in this way, push aside the contextual dimension to which it must necessarily make reference' (Lord and Dufort, 1996: 7). This was reflected in Chapter 5 where we highlighted how many professionals become so concerned with the therapeutic goals of empowerment strategies that they neglect the socio-political goals. Hence participation in itself becomes the target and changes achieved by it become incidental. Yet if this leads to little change it may well be extremely frustrating to the service users drawn into consultation and participation – as was again illustrated in Chapter 5 when discussing service users' experience of both user committees in day centres and involvement in wider planning forums.

Such differences in expectations are also reflected in different perceptions of the 'success and failure' of consultation and participation initiatives. A social work professional involved in a major consultation exercise over the future of mental health services in one UK authority has written of it as a genuine success for user involvement because of the extensive involvement of service users in the processes that led to its report and recommendations (Coe, 1992). Yet our own extended contacts with some of the service users involved reveals a different picture. On the one hand they gained from that involvement and felt that they did have some influence on its final recommendations. However, not only did they have reservations about some aspects of other participants' behaviour towards them, but they were considerably frustrated and potentially disempowered by the fact that they felt uninvolved in the consideration of the recommendations in the policy arena and particularly by what they perceived as the limited degree of change that the exercise created.

Another consistent theme to emerge concerns the limitations placed by simply grafting some form of user involvement onto existing structures. One issue highlighted in our survey among principal officers in social services departments was that this inevitably meant that often such involvement could only be reactive (Bowl, 1996a). Hence it took place after general plans had been drafted or detailed proposals for specific initiatives developed. Managers and practitioners had, therefore, already generated commitments to the ideas, making them harder to affect. Members of user committees in our in-depth study made the related point that they were carefully limited in the areas over which they had an influence – in particular they had no influence over resources dedicated to staffing, which they saw as critical in creating any real change (ibid.). This is also mirrored in the frustration experienced by service users in Milewa's research when the consultation forums they belonged to were unable to even get a response from managers to many proposals concerning funding priorities (Milewa, 1997). Indeed Milewa argues that the exercise revealed just how difficult it is for service users to gain a voice within the health sector – because, despite the rhetoric of change, continuing managerial and clinical hegemony means that it is not necessary to account for the weight attached to the views of local people (including service users) *vis-à-vis* those of other stakeholders or how these ideas have been weighed against other considerations. Furthermore, the role of such consultations is to inform purchasers but purchasing is not the transparently ordered rational process implied in policy. In reality, it reflects bureaucratic needs for continuity and convenience, ideological assumptions and pragmatic needs to sustain a range of required services.

The broader context

In Chapter 5 we argued that one factor that made it difficult to gauge the impact of the users/survivors movement on the public was that, although legislation and policy changes suggested a degree of endorsement of its ideas and philosophies, other public protests and apparent popular support for more restrictive legislation implies equally some resistance to them. Similarly, even though we identify positive changes in services in response to the initiatives of service users, we also have to recognise that other forces have an influence on the way services are shaped and hence serve to limit the extent to which service users are able to produce change. In particular, lobby groups representing the different interests and concerns of carers, such as NSF, and alliances of professionals and carers, such as the Zito Trust have been successful in influencing the thinking of policy makers.

Furthermore, one of the achievements of those lobby groups has been to bolster enthusiasm for biological psychiatry. Despite the existence of 'an extensive body of theory and research which charts the ways that social inequalities... are causally linked to the despair, distress, and confusion that is named mental illness' (Williams and Lindley, 1996: 3), that evidence remains marginalised within many training programmes and goes unreflected in the practice of most mental health professionals. Just as happened earlier in the USA (McLean, 1995), the search for the biological roots of mental distress and new chemical means for suppressing symptoms dominate research programmes in mental health. Perhaps this in itself might be seen partly as a reaction to the greater lay control of and challenge to professional autonomy implied in the very legislative and practice changes that have encouraged user involvement. Certainly its effect is to reinforce the idea that mental health is best left to the scientifically-informed experts. As such, it serves to undermine the idea that service users have an important contribution to the shaping and provision of help.

Nor, even if we doubt the notion that we live in a 'post-modern' society that is somehow qualitatively different from what preceded it, can we deny that in recent years many of the traditional affiliations that gave us the basis for our identity have been weakened. In turn the search for new coherent identities, has led to a reinforcement of the tendency to distance ourselves from those perceived as different and to the renewed location of people in mental distress as the 'other'. This has both fed into and drawn from the development of an increased sense of fear that has seen a demonisation of those experiencing mental distress and the exaggeration of the dangers to public safety created by decarceration policies.

In such a context just how much could mental health services be expected to change in response to the demands of the service user movement? Change is also not likely to happen overnight. We have argued that professional attitudes and orientation are important yet it would be unreasonable to expect these to change immediately, particularly as we have not yet seen the impact of changes in patterns of training that have begun to reflect the influence of the movement. Further changing public perceptions is also going to be critical and yet that process has barely begun. Overall, in assessing the impact of the users/survivors movement, it may be useful to borrow the perspective of resource mobilisation theory which suggests that the success of a social movement rests on:

1. the activities of the movement in pursuing its goals
2. the organisational bases of support
3. the political climate.

Studies of individual coalitions have shown how important the political climate is (Nelson, 1994). In a political climate dominated by risk aversion and a perception of an increased threat to public safety from those experiencing severe psychological distress, despite evidence to the contrary (Taylor and Gunn, 1999), it is perhaps therefore not surprising that as yet major changes have not been wrought in the UK mental health system. Also while the users/survivors movement has made significant steps forward, it does not yet have the solid network of self-help and self-advocacy groups with consistent demands and strategies that is evident in the USA. Furthermore there is little immediate hope of a significant growth in expenditure. In its absence, the development of services more attuned to movement demands is only going to be achieved by switching resources, re-shaping existing services. Given the climate of resistance identified above, this will be difficult whatever the level of activity the movement can generate. However, resource mobilisation theory also outlines how the success of a movement can be gauged by:

1. changes in public policy
2. changes in who is involved in making policy and the processes by which it is evolved
3. changes in the allocation of resources
4. changes in collective consciousness
5. the development of organisational structures that permit further mobilisation.

The ultimate target of the UK users/survivors movement may well be changes in policy and resource distribution and as yet our evidence suggests relatively little change. Nonetheless, we hope that in Chapters 4, 5 and 6 we have demonstrated that the movement has achieved some change in consciousness, made significant steps forward in building an organisational base and gained access to decision-making forums, putting themselves in a position to have a significant input in shaping the future of mental health services. In Chapter 7 we set the prospects of realising that potential within the context of a more detailed consideration of the literature on new social movements.

7

Social movements and social change

Our aim in this chapter is to step outside the mental health policy arena to consider the place which mental health service user movements might occupy in the context of broader shifts in the nature of social action and the contribution that may make to social change. We argued in Chapter 1 that empowerment needs to be addressed within a broad social context and here we offer an analysis of user self-organisation which can address ways in which this wider concept of empowerment may be achieved. In this analysis our perspective is on the movement as a whole, rather than on individual user groups or specific examples of user-led projects, although we will use these to illustrate how specific groups or projects may be contributing to a broader design. In order to address user self-organisation from this perspective we apply analyses developed to understand what have been termed 'new social movements' and to relate such analyses to post-structural analyses of power relations. We start by providing a brief introduction to new social movements (NSMs) and theories that have sought to account for their development, strategies and impact.

What are new social movements?

The notion of a 'new' social movement implies the existence of an 'old' (or old type) movement. In an article originally published in 1951 Blumer defines social movements generally as: 'collective enterprises to establish a new order of life. They have their inception in a condition of unrest, and derive their motive power on one hand from dissatisfaction with the current form of life, and on the other hand, from wishes and hopes for a new scheme of living' (Blumer, 1995). Blumer goes on to discuss a range of social movements which most recent analysts would separate into old and new movements: the labour movement, the youth movement, the women's movement and the peace movement. Most NSM theorists

134

would now locate the labour movement as an example of an 'old' movement to be distinguished from the other three 'new' movements which are not based in class divisions. They would also be likely to add the environmental movement, the gay and lesbian movement and sometimes the disabled people's movement and movements based in ethnic identity as examples of new movements.

The assumption that the binary distinction between 'new' and 'old' reflects an absolute distinction between different types of social movements has been questioned by a number of theorists. For example, Cohen (1985) suggests that it may be more appropriate to talk of 'contemporary' social movements to refer to movements which have emerged in the particular social context of late twentieth-century western society and which thus need to be understood by reference to the particular historical and social location within which they operate. However, we would then need to account for contemporary versions of movements such as the women's movement which are not 'new' (in terms of only having emerged during the latter part of the twentieth century), but which may have undergone significant change as a result both of the changing context within which they operate, and perhaps as a result of the achievement or partial achievement of early aims.

The debate about precise distinctions between new and old movements may not be a particularly fruitful avenue to explore for our purposes. However, it is helpful to look more closely at analyses of contemporary movements which have sought to locate them within broader theorisations of the nature of contemporary society in order to reflect on the goals and characteristics of the mental health users/survivors movement.

Melucci (1985) has suggested that a shared identity 'constructed and negotiated through a repeated process of "activation" of social relationships connecting the actors' distinguishes 'new' from 'old' social movements. The emphasis is on agency, rather than class location, and as Melucci suggests, identities are created and re-created not simply by 'being', but through action within such movements. Thus the objectives of NSMs are not solely or primarily concerned with redistribution, structural revolution or reform, as in the case of class-based movements. They are also concerned with cultural and expressive objectives based in identity formation or consciousness raising (Cohen, 1985). The overarching objective can be expressed as one of transformation rather than restructuring. The means by which this is to be achieved is through a transformation of the values and meanings predominating in what has been variously termed the 'post-industrial' or 'post-modern' world.

Key features of the post-industrial society are that it is characterised by fragmentation and uncertainty. Empirically, the structuring of society that led to people deriving their collective identities from their employment and the position this occupied within the economic and social hierarchies defining social class, is considered to have broken down. It is considered to have been replaced by a multiplicity of identities through which people locate themselves in their social world. Theoretically, the certainty of grand theories and meta-narratives and the control they offer over the possibility of progress has been undermined, and all forms of knowledge have been subject to the critique of relativism. In that context, the forms of political action which can give expression to experience of oppression or dissent are unlikely to be grounded in class-based mass political movements, but in single issue action or in the politics of identity. The aim is not a redistribution of wealth, but to gain control over the discourse within which lives are constructed.

These transformative rather than redistributive goals affect the nature of the social action within which contemporary movements are engaged. Contemporary social movements adopt a variety of forms of action which are not based in traditional forms of political participation – such as party membership or political lobbying – but which utilise a range of sub- and counter-cultural strategies such as festivals, the celebration of alternative life styles, consciousness raising and direct action. Melucci (1985) describes the goals of NSMs as symbolic and cultural, concerned with the meaning and orientation of social action and providing a vision for future models of social interaction. Cohen (1985) suggests: 'they target the social domain of "civil society" rather than the economy or state, raising issues concerned with the democratisation of structures of everyday life and focusing on forms of communication and collective identity' (ibid.: 667). Thus the forms of action in which NSMs are engaged themselves express the values they seek to promote.

NSMs are themselves diverse. Diversity and heterogeneity are key themes within the theorisation of contemporary society and social and political relations (for example Bock and James, 1992; Phillips, 1993; Sibley, 1995; Seidman, 1998). Collective action through which such diversity is expressed is unlikely to conform to a single model. One difference among contemporary movements has been variously expressed as a distinction between instrumental and expressive movements, or strategy oriented and identity oriented movements (for example Cohen, 1985;

Kriesi *et al.*, 1995). Elsewhere we have suggested it is important to distinguish identity and interest-based movements (Barnes, 1999c). A pragmatic way of understanding this distinction is to ask who can become a member of the movement. Potentially anyone, regardless of personal characteristics or social circumstances, can take part in the peace movement or the environmental movement. In other instances membership is exclusive to those accepting or adopting a specific identity: lesbians, gay men, disabled people or feminists, for example. Kreisi *et al.* (op. cit.) have related such differences to inner or outer directed orientations and to the level of activity and volume of participation evident among movements.

Scott (1990) has suggested a potentially huge range of 'identities' (including that of animal lover or rate-payer) which might form the basis of social movement mobilisation. This is not particularly helpful as a basis for distinguishing one-off, goal-directed action (such as a rent strike) which does not lead to any lasting basis for organising, from social movements with broad social change objectives. Phillips (1993, 1995) has argued the need to distinguish temporary from intensely felt identities based in common cultures and common languages as a basis for a new 'politics of presence' appropriate to a new pluralism.

The radical critique of meanings and values offered by NSMs has provided a challenge not only to social policies and practices, but to the rational scientific basis of knowledge production. Referring to the American context Seidman describes this aspect of new social movements as follows:

> These new social movements created new subjects of knowledge (African-Americans, women, lesbians and gay men) and new knowledges. Socially positioned as oppressed, Blacks, gays, women, lesbians and Chicanos developed new perspectives on knowledge, society and politics. The dominant knowledges in American public culture were criticized as reflecting the standpoint and interests of White Europeans, men and heterosexuals. Black nationalists, feminists, gay liberationists, and lesbian feminists produced social perspectives that were said to express their distinctive social reality: Afrocentrism, feminism, lesbian and gay or Queer theory. (1998: 254)

This challenge to the dominance of Enlightenment thought offered by contemporary social movements has been addressed from a number of perspectives. For example, Harding (1991) has argued the necessity for a feminist science in the sphere not only of the social sciences but also of the natural sciences. This in order to challenge the 'weak objectivity' of knowledge produced only from the perspectives of elite groups. Wainwright (1994) locates the place of social movements as agents of social change in the 'shared interrogation of their everyday knowledge' (ibid.: 105) and emphasises the connection between knowledge and social action. Altman (1994) has identified the challenge to the dominance of biomedical models of disease and disease control offered by action from within the gay community in relation to AIDS. His question 'Who Owns AIDS?' mirrors that asked by Figert in relation to PMS (see Chapter 4).

The theoretical underpinning of this analysis of the link between social movements and contested knowledge comes from Foucault's analysis of the exercise of power through dominant discourses (see Chapter 1). It also reflects the work of the critical realist school of social theorists and the cultural studies tradition within sociology. Each of these takes an anti-positivist stance and views knowledge production as socially situated. They come within what has been described as the 'theoretical stance' or 'style of work' known as social constructionism (Velody and Williams, 1998). But as Wainwright and others (for example Shakespeare, 1998) have argued, social constructionism can comprise a political strategy as well as a theoretical explanation. The goal of creating new meanings and new understandings from the experiences of marginalised and oppressed groups is intimately tied in with political goals of broad social change.

User and survivor movements as contemporary social movements

As we have indicated, the disabled people's movement is now included in some discussions of NSMs. Disability theorists and activists have undertaken such an analysis, but more general theorists have also referred to the disability movement within discussions of identity-based social movements and political action (for example Oliver, 1990; Shakespeare, 1993, 1998; Campbell and Oliver, 1996; Lister, 1997). In some cases these analyses have reflected on the multiple identities which comprise individual and collective experiences of disability and which reflect the diverse standpoints from which different social movement theorists and activists have sought to mobilise. For example, Morris (1989) has argued the importance of a feminist perspective within the disability movement, while Corbett (1994) has discussed the relationship between disability politics and gay politics.

Mental health users/survivors movements have received rather less attention within this theoretical framework. Indeed, as we argue elsewhere in this book there have been few studies of the movement as a whole and much of the evidence about its nature and impact derives from small-scale studies and activists' accounts. Rogers and Pilgrim's (1991) study is one exception. This draws on Offe's (1984) analysis of NSMs in order to account for the emergence of the mental health users/survivors movement and to suggest likely future prospects for the movement. They locate the movement's emergence within the failure of traditional political parties to represent adequately the interests of marginalised social groups and to the permanent crisis within a welfare state increasingly unable to satisfy the needs of different groups. Thus, they argue, the 'chronicity' of 'psychiatric patients' who have lengthy periods in contact with health service professionals is conducive to their politicisation because they become very aware of the inadequacies of the welfare system. This was given added impetus by the advent of consumerism during the 1980s and the fact that sympathetic managers were able to legitimate their support for user groups within mental health services by reference to the need to listen to users' views (see Chapter 3). However, Rogers and Pilgrim suggest that the movement is weakened by being defined by the services with which participants have contact, and by the stigmatising diagnostic labels assigned within that system:

> This has the effect of focusing their [users/survivors] remit of demands on the narrow agenda of clinical services and diverting energy from wider social and material provision which is recognised in principle as being important (for example jobs, adequate housing, non-medicalised support networks). Indeed one of the respondents identified this as a vulnerability within the movement. This also suggests that the identity of mental patient is indeed bound up with service providers, giving partial support to the social constructivist position mentioned earlier and casting doubt on the success of the MHUM [Mental Health User Movement] in transcending medical discourse. (ibid.: 147)

This potential danger or weakness has been alluded to in our earlier discussions of the dilemmas posed for user groups in deciding whether to work with the grain of the mental health system, or to remain separate and offer a radical critique or alternative from outside the system. However, our description of the range of activity and strategies evident within the movement as a whole suggests there may be a more optimistic scenario for the movement. Before we go on to consider the evidence that is available concerning this broad impact it is necessary to go beyond the analysis offered by Rogers and Pilgrim to draw on a wider range of thinking about the nature of NSMs and how the user/survivor movement might locate itself within this sphere.

Contested identities

We suggested above that it is possible to draw a distinction between movements which coalesce around an issue (such as environmentalism or the peace movement) and those based in collective identities (such as the women's movement and the user/survivor movement). However, the notion of a unitary identity which can capture the diverse range of experiences is itself problematic. During the 1980s the women's movement became increasingly subject to critique from black women and working-class women as being a predominately white, middle-class movement not least because it failed to recognise the broad range of experiences it sought to incorporate within the category of 'women'. It also drew criticism because it assumed the priority assigned to a gender identity when, for example, black women might prioritise the experience of racism and thus action with black men rather then with white women as a means of challenging oppression (for example Davis, 1981).

There are other problems with the notion of identity. We have argued elsewhere (for example Barnes and Shardlow, 1996; Barnes, 1999c) that the articulation of their own identity by users and survivors is a key goal of the user movement. We have also suggested that the stigmatised identity of 'mental patient' has led many to emphasise the normality of psychological distress and to link this to the common experience of stress with which most people are familiar. This has been particularly important to user groups seeking to counteract the impact of media images which link madness to violence and have thus contributed to an increasing emphasis on control within mental health policy. Developing a sense of shared experience and a shared identity has been important as a basis for self-help and the creation of environments within which people can be confident that the impact of their distress is understood. It has also been a basis from which competence can be demonstrated and both medical and lay discourses relating to the nature of 'the mentally disordered' can be challenged.

However, the notion of 'normality' or 'ordinariness' can also be problematic. 'Ordinary life' can contribute to the development of the psychological distress experienced by many people, particularly when 'ordinary' life also comprises the experience of racism or sexual abuse (for example Campbell, 1988; Fraser, 1989). A perceived deviation from 'normal' gender roles can be cited as evidence of mental disorder and normative assumptions about appropriate expressions of happiness, fear, anger, sadness and other emotions can affect clinical perceptions of 'recovery' (see below). We have discussed in Chapter 4 how the category 'mental health service user' or 'survivor' has needed to be differentiated if empowerment strategies are to be effective in enabling women and black people to empower themselves in response to the multiple experiences of oppression.

For many disabled people a fundamental goal of the disability movement is to reject the normalising project of medical interventions such as conductive education and to assert the value of difference (for example Oliver, 1996; Davis, 1995). There have also been reactions against a 'blurring of the boundaries' between sanity and madness and an attempt to re-assert the difference or otherness represented by madness. Writing in *OpenMind*, the MIND journal, Perkins called for an embracing of 'mad pride' stating:

> For therapists, allies, those who have not been defined as mad, notions of distress remove the discomfort of difference, create the illusion of understanding and shared experience. The sane can rest secure in the knowledge that their own distress affords them understanding and insight into madness as though it were simply an extension of their own experience. They do not have to confront their own lack of knowing. (Perkins, 1999: 6)

Similar attempts to reclaim madness are evident in groups and networks such as 'MadNation' (http://www.madnation.org). One contributor to this website stressed the reality of the distinction between survivors and 'normal' people in terms of the response received from others:

> There is a degree of exposure in the lives of psych. survivors that so-called normal people never have to deal with. If you're normal you can yell when you're hurt, throw a plate in a fit of anger, or curse and swear until the anger runs out of you. If you're a psych. patient in a hospital such behaviour gets you held down in four- or five-point restraints while nurses plunge hypodermics into your body unheeding of your screams. (http://www.madnation.org/news/rohmer.htm)

Millett's book *The Loony Bin Trip* illustrates one person's experience of the results of being declared 'mentally ill' in terms of the way in which other people, including close friends, responded to her. She reflects on the problematic distinction between sanity and madness, but finds these concepts considerably more attractive than those of mental illness, psychosis or disorders.

> We do not lose our minds, even 'mad' we are neither insane nor sick. Reason gives way to fantasy – both are mental activities, both productive. The mind goes on working, speaking a different language, making its own perceptions, designs, symmetrical or asymmetrical; it works. We only have to lose our fear of its workings. (ibid.: 315)

There is little evidence that this assertion of a mad identity is widespread within the mental health user movement. However, it is possible to draw parallels not only with disabled people's rejection of normalisation, but also with recent developments within the gay and lesbian movement which have sought to reclaim language which has been used to abuse and stigmatise in the context of a resistance to the normalising process. Queer theorists and activists have reacted against the liberal, rights-based and normalising streams of thought and action within the mainstream gay and lesbian movement. They have challenged the notion of a unitary gay identity arguing that any attempt to define ever more specific and multiple identities (such as black lesbian) has an inevitable exclusionary effect. But rather than attempting to define identity on the basis of difference or opposition the focus for analysis should be on the way in which binary opposition categories (such as heterosexual/homosexual) structure core modes of thought and affect not only the minority directly involved, but the whole social order (Seidman, 1998).

Applying a similar analysis to the mental health context would not imply an argument for the blurring of the boundaries between those defined as sane or mad rejected by Perkins. It would constitute a plea to understand the way in which notions of sanity and madness construct social relations throughout society. From this perspective, the goals of 'mad theorists' (if such were to identify themselves) might be less concerned with securing the rights of those defined as 'mentally disordered' but with addressing the way in which the category of mental disorder is socially produced and the impact this has on social practices and policies. We would suggest that Millet's autobiographical account seeks to do just this by exploring the way in which an ascription of a psychiatric diagnosis was seen to provide legitimation not only for unwanted interventions from medical professionals, but also for the watchful supervision of friends. This perspective is little theorised within the user or survivor movement. However, many of the arguments being advanced by users about the way legislation to force people to become recipients of services and treatments is considered legitimate in the case of mental illness but not physical illness, are also based in such an analysis of the binary distinction between madness and sanity and the way this operates to discriminate and oppress 'the mentally disordered'.

Making links

There are other ways in which the mental health users/survivors movements can be considered to constitute a broader social movement which has moved beyond being defined by participants' relationships with particular services. Activists within the mental health users/survivors movement have contributed to a questioning of fundamental societal values as well as seeking more sympathetic and responsive mental health services. One example of this is Davey's analyses of the links between physical, social and economic environment and mental health (for example Davey, 1994, 1999). This analysis is important because of the direction it suggests for action to enable people who have used mental health services to become more empowered within their personal lives and the communities in which they live. It also identifies the way in which environmental circumstances can contribute to the developments of psychological distress. It thus makes significant connections between the value base of the environmental movement and the empowerment strategies of the user movement:

> Danger from traffic is another example of environmental influences damaging adult–child relations. The need to be constantly under supervision limits the development of children, infringing on their independence and autonomy, perhaps creating a tendency of parents to 'over-control' which we have already seen to be so damaging – and which could lead to 'High EE' relationships. In Nottingham, at the time of writing, there is a discussion about what can be done to improve long-term community mental health in response to the government's 'Aiming for Health Campaign'. The Nottingham Health Authority proposals include a need for traffic calming and safe play areas for children. (Davey, 1994: 193)

Davey's analysis, and the practical initiatives flowing from this in the Ecoworks project in Nottingham, explicitly challenge a definition of empowerment strategies within the mental health user movement based in identities as mental patients. Indeed Davey has argued that it is necessary to go beyond those identities if any real empowerment is to be achieved.

A wider perspective is also evident in the 'Strategies for Living' programme and the 'Knowing our Own Minds' survey led by service users and survivors at the Mental Health Foundation (Faulkner, 1997). The survey demonstrated the extent to which people had gone beyond mainstream mental health services in order to develop strategies to deal with their distress. It argued the need for a holistic perspective on mental health in order to take account not only of mental, but also spiritual, physical and emotional aspects of people's lives. Both the process and the outcome of this work demonstrate the extent to which the user and survivor movement has moved beyond 'consumer' identities focused solely on achieving changes within the mental health system and struggling to transcend the medical discourse. The role of users in creating new knowledge about both effective survival strategies and the limitations of a medical discourse in providing solutions to severe psychological distress, point to this. The survey results also indicate that there has been some success in inserting alternative therapies into mainstream services. Over half of those receiving alternative or complementary therapies such as art/creative therapies, physical therapies (for example massage, acupuncture, osteopathy), exercise/postural therapies, dietary and natural supplements, hobbies and leisure activities and talking treatments, had received these from NHS or social services providers. However, it is likely that the majority of instances referred to some form of counselling and therapy service and there is evidence from this survey and elsewhere that such treatments are unequally available to those who might seek them (NHSE, 1996).

Such developments suggest that a view of the users/survivors movement as defined by diagnostic labels and relationships with services is incomplete and that the movement is playing a wider role in the process of identity negotiation and the transformation of cultural values and meanings.

Social movements and social change strategies

One aspect of NSM theory concerns the forms of action in which such movements engage and the difference between these and traditional forms of political action. The political and cultural objectives of new social movements relate not only to the ends to be secured, but also to the processes through which social, political and cultural life is conducted. Some movements have included an objective of opening existing political processes to a more diverse set of interests and a broader range of actors. An obvious example of this would be the objective of electing more women and more black people as members of parliament. However, such an objective is not seen as an end in itself, but a means towards transforming the democratic dialogue. Rather than external lobbyists acting behind the scenes and seeking to secure specific, and often narrow, benefits deriving from individual or group self-interests, participation can change the nature of the discussion itself (Phillips, 1993; Wainwright, 1994). Not only are previously excluded participants potentially in a position to be taken seriously when speaking on behalf of the group they 'represent', they are also in a position to influence the perception and behaviour of dominant groups through dialogue and example. Bringing difference into mainstream political life (and into social life more broadly) has the capacity to challenge assumptions, increase awareness of injustice and transform the terms in which public debate is conducted.

Nevertheless, the political objectives of new social movements have usually been seen to oppose existing political structures, and thus participation in the existing mechanisms of government may not be a priority. Indeed the unconventional forms of political action pursued by new social movements are seen to present a challenge in themselves to the dominant political order (Dalton *et al.*, 1990). A distinction is drawn between neo-corporatist approaches to influence through which pressure groups achieve the status of recognised and legitimate participants in the process of governing (as in the days when trades union negotiators enjoyed beer and sandwiches at Number 10), and new social movements which intentionally remain outside such institutionalised frameworks. Thus civil disobedience, planned protest and direct action are seen to be the hallmarks of the political style of new social movements, while internal organisation is correspondingly fluid with few formal roles, shifting membership and no hierarchy (Dalton *et al.*, 1990; Oliver, 1990; Scott 1990).

Phillips (1993) cites examples of attempts within radical left local authorities to secure a voice for excluded or marginalised groups – primarily women and ethnic minorities – which were undermined because there were no procedures through which such communities could elect their own spokespeople. Each group was dependent on the patronage of the authority and to secure this had to argue that the deprivation experienced by its members was greater than that experienced by other groups.

She uses this (and other examples) to argue for a model of pluralist politics which involves neither competition between excluded groups based on sectarian loyalties, nor an essentially private retreat to separate spaces in which difference can be pursued for its own sake.

Her argument provides an important perspective on the participatory project evident in the objectives which have been articulated by disabled people. Oliver (1990) has constructed a typology of disability organisations which traces developments from self-help to political action, with the common theme being that of disabled people defining and participating in seeking their own solutions to their problems. While control of the movement by disabled people is fundamental to the challenge being offered, this is not seen to represent a retreat into entirely separatist action. Oliver writes of the movement 'crossing the borderline' between state and civil society by engaging in service development and representation within the state political apparatus, as well as opening up possibilities of co-operation with other excluded groups through a common analysis of oppression.

Nevertheless, such action is founded upon and defined by disabled people's self-identification and underpinned by an ideological challenge to medical models of disability previously accepted as the norm. The social model of disability is more than an argument for an accessible environment. It can be considered to represent Touraine's fifth type of social conflict: 'whose stake is *the social control of the main cultural patterns*, that is, of the patterns through which our relationships with the environment are normatively organized' (1985: 754–5).

Autonomy is both an individual and a collective aim and a method of action for social movements. Reclaiming the right to define themselves and their own problems is a prerequisite for attaining other objectives (Melucci, 1985). Scott (1990) traces the link between developing personal autonomy (for example through personal consciousness raising), through the extension of personal and group autonomy by means of the assertion of social and political rights and opposition to discrimination, to what he refers to as the 'autonomy of struggle' – an insistence on fighting the movement's own struggle without interference from elsewhere. While personal consciousness raising may be of particular significance for those engaged in identity groups, activists and analysts considering different movements assert the importance of moving from the development of personal autonomy to the achievement of collective consciousness and action.

The political nature of personal experiences of mental distress, and of professional/client relationships within the mental health system, have been identified as sites for action by the user movement. The literature of both the mental health and disability movements includes personal statements which describe experiences which have resulted in decisions to participate in these movements as well as forming the basis for an analysis of the challenges to be overcome (for example Chamberlin, 1988; French, 1993). Cultural expression through poetry, theatre and the visual arts is increasingly being recognised as a means not only of exploring personal experiences of madness and the treatment meted out to those so designated, but also as a strategy for change.

As we have seen there are differences within the mental health user movement about the merits of operating entirely outside the local or national state apparatus. In practical terms this has often meant a distinction between groups which are prepared to work with professional 'allies' and those which reject all professional authority. Once again, the key theme is that of the active participation and self-definition of people who have been schooled to adopt a passive, 'patient' role. Participation within forums from which users have previously been excluded is an end in itself. It also offers a means of transforming the dialogic process and the nature of the policy produced within official decision-making forums.

Nevertheless, Rogers and Pilgrim's (1991) suggestion that one of the weaknesses of the mental health user movement has been in relying on the support of professional sympathisers needs to be heeded. Jensen and Froestad (1988) identified a similar danger of co-option in their study of client organisations in Norway:

> In addition to the general problems tied to poverty of resources the clients suffer from lack of self-confidence which is often a result of a long-lasting career as a client. An organisation of the powerless will also be more susceptible to influence. This creates dangers for the growing of oligarchy and different kinds of co-optation from professions, political organisations, bureaucracies and companies. (ibid.: 87)

However, other social movement theorists have suggested that movements develop within contexts that provide opportunities to transform the potential for mobilisation into action (Tarrow, 1998). Tarrow identifies the following dimensions of the contexts in which social movements are most likely to emerge:

1. the opening of access to participation for new actors;
2. the evidence of political realignment within the polity;

3. the appearance of influential allies;
4. emerging splits within the elite;
5. a decline in the state's capacity or will to repress dissent (ibid.: 76).

This suggests that the conditions within which a social movement can grow are also potentially those in which contention is unlikely to lead to repression: 'Challengers are encouraged to take collective action when they have allies who can act as friends in court, as guarantors against repression, or as acceptable negotiators on their behalf' (ibid.: 79). Such conditions could also be read as facilitating co-option.

In Chapter 3 we quoted Conlan arguing that the user movement needed to take the risks of working within the system in order to reap the rewards of the benefits that could accrue from this. Not all have been happy to take that risk. There are also dilemmas for social movements which achieve some success in acceptance of their objectives and which find themselves with opportunities to implement their ideas through practical projects. Longer established movements than the user/survivor movement have confronted such dilemmas. For example, Lovenduski and Randall (1993) discuss how those involved in the women's refuge movement faced dilemmas of both principle and organisation when statutory authorities started to incorporate approaches originally developed in opposition to existing practices adopted by local authorities, the police and other agencies concerned with domestic violence. Similarly, those involved in the establishment of Women's Therapy Centres have been faced with compromise in order to gain acceptance for their ideas by statutory agencies (Barnes and Maple, 1992: 151–4), and a need to adopt different organisational strategies when seeking to provide services directly (Sturdy, 1987). The reluctance of UK mental health users/survivors movement groups to take on service provision responsibilities reflects an awareness of the constraints such responsibilities can impose on oppositional action and proactive campaigning.

Self-interest or social change?

As we have seen above, ends and means are interconnected in the strategies of social movements. But who benefits from the changes which may be secured? In previous chapters we have discussed evidence of the impact on users/survivors and on the mental health system. Can any broader social value be deduced from their activities?

Dalton *et al.* (1990) contrast the collective goods which new social movements seek to achieve with the logic of self-interested action which the rational choice model takes as a basic precept. Barton (1993) has suggested that 'an understanding of the plight of vulnerable people gives some crucial insights into the nature of society'. Harding's arguments, concerning the significance of feminism and perspectives deriving from the experiences of other marginalised groups in pure as well as social science, provide another perspective on this. She argues that 'strong objectivity' necessary to good science depends on the inclusion of perspectives which can only come from those who do not occupy positions where self-interest demands adherence to the status quo:

> If the community of 'qualified' researchers and critics systematically excludes, for example, all African Americans and women of all races, and if the larger culture is stratified by race and gender and lacks powerful critiques of this stratification, it is not plausible to imagine that racist and sexist interests and values would be identified within a community of scientists composed entirely of people who benefit – intentionally or not – from institutional racism and sexism. (Harding, 1991: 143)

Similar arguments have been made concerning the contribution feminist perspectives are making to both the concept and practice of a citizenship which includes the: 'cluster of activities, values, ways of thinking and ways of doing things which have long been associated with women' (James, 1992). Barton makes similar points about the contribution of disabled people's struggles to the development of citizenship in a way which extends this influence beyond the interests solely of disabled people:

> Establishing effective social relations is seen as integral to the disability rights movement's efforts for radical change. This is a challenge to the dominance of possessive individualism and the ways in which market criteria influence the form in which self-actualisation is packaged as a commodity in modern society. (Barton, 1993: 243)

If the perspectives of marginalised groups are significant as a means of knowing the world in all its diversity, and if the participation of excluded or marginalised groups is a necessary condition for the establishment of social relations which reinforce the humanity rather than objectification of individuals, then the struggles of those groups have benefits beyond the interests of their members.

Scott suggests that successful movements have a significant impact on attitudes and policies. This implies the eventual disappearance of successful groups:

> 'Success' takes the form of integrating previously excluded issues and groups into the 'normal' political process. If there is a telos of social movement activity then it is the normalization of previously exotic issues and groups. Success is thus quite compatible with, and indeed overlaps, the disappearance of the movement as a movement. (Scott, 1990: 10–11)

It could be argued that since a key objective of the users/survivors movement is to remove the stigma and oppression attached to the experience of severe psychological distress, the 'normalization of exotic groups' is part of their purpose. So, is the transformative project of new social movements one which is in the interests of their members, or more broadly, those sharing key characteristics with members, or can such projects be understood to have a universal relevance? This question is addressed by Hewitt (1993) who argues that social movements are concerned with universal needs and hence cannot be understood as narrow interest groups.

In Chapter 1 we drew on Doyal and Gough's (1991) discussion of autonomy as a universal need and considered how perceptions of impaired autonomy contributed to the disempowerment of people diagnosed with mental illness. Doyal and Gough's argument for the objectivity of such universal needs is based on the necessity of social participation as a means of avoiding harm. The satisfaction of needs is thus a prerequisite for survival without serious harm within the social world. Their discussion of these basic needs is directly related to both physical disability and mental illness (Figure 7.1).

This suggests an immediate relevance to an analysis of the collective objectives of disabled people's movements and users/survivors movements. Such objectives can be understood as being concerned with overcoming the particular restrictions consequent on the experience of impairment and mental distress within a society which disables those who do not conform to physical and mental normality. The achievement of such objectives is necessary if those who are disabled are to achieve the participation necessary for social survival. There are two reasons why this has relevance to those who do not identify themselves as disabled or as psychologically distressed:

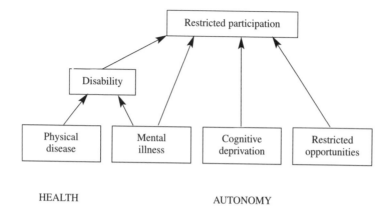

Figure 7.1   The relation between participation, health and autonomy
Source: Doyal and Gough, 1991: 171

1. Physical impairment and severe psychological distress could be experienced by anyone during the course of their life. Thus, everyone is a potential beneficiary of action designed to challenge the disempowerment which can result from this.

2. The systematic exclusion of particular groups leading to their inability to survive without serious harm is a substantial indictment of the human rights record of a society. In material terms this creates a sub-class of 'welfare dependants' who are placed in a position of having to receive rather than to contribute to social, cultural and economic life.

The evidence Doyal and Gough present is at a macro-level designed to compare the performance of states in meeting basic needs of their populations. An analysis of the interaction between user groups and local decision-making processes about welfare policies and services contributes to an understanding of the means by which new social movements can affect such macro-level outcomes, as well as an understanding of the nature of their collective objectives.

Doyal and Gough's analysis also further demonstrates the link between what might be considered cultural or ideological objectives (for example 'autonomy'), and those which make practical demands on the state for action. Thus while: 'The new problems have to do with quality of life, equal rights, individual self-realization, participation and human rights' (Habermas, 1987: 392), their resolution is likely to reside both in the action of groups operating within civil society, and the interaction between such groups and the state designed to achieve concrete ends, including changes in the way in which state services are provided. In the course of such action the pursuit of individual autonomy becomes balanced by the idea and experience of solidarity in the movement; and new images and slogans can reinforce the development of positive identities to be substituted for derogatory or patronising ones (Scott, 1990). Means and ends start to coalesce and hence looking for outcomes solely in evidence about shifts in policy or service provision fails to reflect the significance of the movement as a whole.

Conclusion

How might we relate this analysis to the conceptual discussion of empowerment in Chapter 1? The Foucauldian analysis of the exercise of power by means of dominant discourses is crucial here. The demonstration of competence in analysis, deliberation and action which user and survivor groups provide, presents a challenge to the association between madness, irrationality and incompetence. At an individual level participants experience this as personal empowerment arising from a process of peer and outsider valuing, while collectively this acts to challenge the categorical connection between severe psychological distress, irrationality and incompetence which underpin the more controlling aspects of mental health policy and practice.

Apart from this, the emergence of users/survivors movements as actors outside the domains of the 'mental health system' and in roles, such as researchers and educators, which challenge the dichotomy of 'user' and 'professional', suggest a potential to address disempowerment within the spheres of civil society as well as in the mental health system. However, the weakness of users/survivors movements in addressing issues of poverty and structural exclusion from the labour market is an indication of limitations of NSMs generally in addressing the real structural inequalities which remain. In the final chapter we suggest what the prospects might be for users/survivors movements to link with other areas of action for social change which may have some impact in these areas.

8

Future prospects

In this final chapter we summarise some of the conclusions which can be drawn from the evidence we have presented throughout this book concerning empowerment and mental health. We also highlight some of the changes that are taking place in social policy at the start of the new millennium and the way in which these are likely to influence the context within which struggles for empowerment will take place. Finally, we reflect on how the nature of education and training for mental health workers and the organisational strategies adopted within their employing agencies can help or hinder empowerment. Our discussion is located primarily within the context of UK developments and refers specifically to changes in policy and infrastructure within UK health and social care services. However, important themes within contemporary thinking on 'welfare' are not restricted to the UK. A focus on social exclusion and social cohesion, and on work as a means of reducing exclusion and achieving cohesion, is evident within North American and European social policy. This provides a new context within which the empowerment struggles of users/survivors are being fought.

The evidence so far

Our analysis of the dimensions of disempowerment in the first chapter of this book demonstrated the terrains within which the struggle for empowerment has to be fought. It also described some of the diverse and contested meanings the concept has attracted. In summary, empowerment can relate to personal growth and development; to increased control over the nature of services received individually and collectively; to the power to define the terms within which dialogue about mental health and mental health policy takes place; and to opportunities to take part in the sphere of civil society on equal terms with anyone else. Thus the contexts within which empowerment is sought include the social relations of everyday life, as well as policies and services intended specifically to address the needs of people experiencing severe psychological distress. Throughout these varying terrains, power is exercised in the course of day-to-day interactions between those deemed 'mad' and those claiming sanity – especially those occupying positions of authority which enable them to define and control the nature of the support to be provided to those in distress. This diffuseness in the way in which power is exercised is one of the reasons why it is so difficult both to achieve and 'measure' shifts in the balance of power.

We have traced examples of resistance from mental health service users to inhumane treatment within the mental health system to the nineteenth century. However, the emergence of anything like a national users/survivors movement, which has the capacity to challenge not only poor treatment within the system but also stigma and exclusion beyond it, is a recent phenomenon both in the UK and elsewhere. It would be unrealistic to expect radical transformations in either the subjective understandings of the general population, or the objective circumstances of those experiencing severe psychological distress within a short time period. As we have also indicated, we need to understand the opportunities and the strategies adopted to pursue social change objectives within the context of a changing policy environment and of broader shifts in social relations. These construct the terms within which a change dialogue can take place. For example, a dialogue constructed as taking place between consumer-oriented providers and service users asserting their rights to have a say in their treatment by reference to Patient's Charter rights, implies one set of strategies and objectives. That conducted between the contested knowledges of professional mental health workers and the expert 'citizen user' implies another (see Barnes, 1999c). The histories of social movements do not suggest a straightforward 'march of progress' towards the achievement of objectives, but rather a story of increasing complexity, diversity and sometimes fragmentation.

During our working lifetime we have observed (and in some ways been part of) a process in which recipients of services have come to occupy positions as contributors to the production of services, the training of workers and the generation of knowledge. We have heard personal testimony of the impact of such experiences on those formerly defined by their position as recipients of services and have observed the challenge that such a role reversal can present to those trained to regard themselves as 'experts' in mental health. As Wallcraft has written:

despite centuries of stigmatisation, the voice of psychiatric survivors is making itself heard in debating chambers, conference halls and training and education establishments. The consciousness-raising and educative work that they are doing, by valuing their own and each others' experience, are making the unthinkable possible. People who had been written off by the medical profession and society, people with labels of schizophrenia and manic depression, and people who had been institutionalised and regarded as unemployable are finding new roles as mental health educators, advocates, organisers of self-help services and consultants to purchasing authorities. Government, professional and voluntary sector bodies are consulting self-advocacy groups and reporting their findings; often commissioning survivors to do the research and writing. For the first time in history, current and former mental patients are breaking their isolation and silence, and speaking out collectively and individually. (Wallcraft, 1996: 188)

In the same article Wallcraft defines 'taking over the asylum' as a process of reclaiming the right to define what asylum means and how it should be experienced by those needing refuge in times of crisis. The process of taking over the institutions through which support, care and perhaps treatment is to be provided to those experiencing severe psychological distress is as much about being able to define the nature of 'the problem' and what are acceptable and appropriate solutions to this, as it is about taking part in decisions about service commissioning strategies or in staff recruitment procedures. Empowerment is as much about achieving recognition for the legitimacy of experiential knowledge as a basis on which decisions about mental health policy and practice should be developed as it is about being able to take part in a day centre user council, or even to enter into contracts to provide user run services.

We share Wallcraft's assessment of the significance of the changes that have taken place in the last 15–20 years. However, we are also cautious about the depth of the transformation that has taken place. First we note how current policy continues to be strongly influenced by stereotypes of the 'mad, bad and dangerous' schizophrenic or psychopath. We also have the evidence of more personal accounts of service users who find themselves involved in a process of compulsory hospital admission, when they thought they were seeking counselling support, or who have been subjected to the indignities of having their underwear and personal items logged and counted during voluntary admission to hospital (accounts from users during the process of preparing for a joint study, between

Birmingham University, NAG, User Voice (Birmingham) and Reflect (Solihull), of users' experiences of compulsion under the 1983 Mental Health Act).

Hence a fundamental shift in the balance of power remains to be achieved. Nonetheless it is unlikely that there will be a radical reversal of the view that users of mental health services should have some say in determining the nature of those services and should have a legitimate place around at least some of the tables at which policy is decided. Also while autonomous user groups may continue to struggle for the resources which will ensure a degree of stability and independence, there is little evidence that users and survivors will not continue to organise and seek to be heard on their own terms – both within the mental health system and in seeking wider recognition and public understanding. We will conclude this chapter by reflecting on the policy and practice context within which such strategies for empowerment are likely to be pursued into the twenty-first century.

Rediscovering inequality and community

Under the Conservative governments of Margaret Thatcher and John Major in the 1980s and early 1990s it became impossible to talk of 'inequalities' in health. The start of the Thatcher years saw the suppression of the *Black Report*, which had been commissioned by a previous Labour government to investigate evidence of health inequalities. Then at the end of the period a major research programme was commissioned by the Economic and Social Research Council which was defined by the deliberately value neutral concept of 'health variations'. One of the earliest actions of the Labour government elected in 1997 was to invite health authorities, in partnership with local authorities and the voluntary, community and private sectors, to bid for 'Health Action Zone' status. Health Action Zones (HAZs) were evidence that the new government was persuaded that improving health could not be achieved solely by the National Health Service. As the originally somewhat vague notion of what a HAZ actually was started to become clearer, as plans were produced and started to be implemented, and as the government pursued its policy agenda for both the NHS and local government, HAZs became a central plank of the government's twin objectives of improving health and *reducing health inequalities*. There was official recognition that 'variations' in health constituted structural inequalities which needed to be addressed by both national and local policy.

Closely related to the objective of reducing health inequalities were those of *increasing social cohesion* and *reducing social exclusion*. The HAZ policy was only one of a number of social policies that focused on the need to 'regenerate' communities. While Margaret Thatcher had declared 'there is no such thing as society', Tony Blair appealed to the moral agency of communities to play an active part in neighbourhood renewal, increasing community safety and addressing the alienation and disaffection of young people (Barnes and Prior, 2000). A concern with the health of civil society and with the generation of the social capital considered necessary, not only to improve the quality of social life but also economic performance, became one of the underpinnings of the 'Third Way' being pursued on both sides of the Atlantic (Putnam, 1993; Giddens, 1998).

The acceptance that health status is closely related to socio-economic status and that action to improve health and reduce health inequalities requires action in the spheres of social, economic, environmental and other public policies represents a major shift in thinking. So too does the recognition that social policies need to address the way people live together within communities. At the time of writing, there is little evidence that the Labour Government will offer wholehearted support to the redistributive welfare policies implied by the weight of evidence now in the public sphere (for example Wilkinson, 1996) and argued for directly by the committee commissioned by the new Labour government to undertake yet another inquiry into health inequalities (Acheson, 1998). However, HAZ, Health Improvement Programmes (HImps) and the White Paper *Saving Lives: Our Healthier Nation* (DoH, 1999) mark an important shift in thinking about the nature of action necessary to reduce inequality in health. They represent a move away from the dominance of the medical model towards action on the social, economic and environmental conditions which create poor health. Thus, for example, health authorities seeking to improve morbidity rates in relation to coronary heart disease (CHD) by investing in more heart transplant surgeons would have been unlikely to achieve HAZ status. Those (such as authorities in the South Yorkshire coalfields), which are targeting action to strengthen primary care teams in deprived areas and to involve local communities in health promotion and the prevention of heart disease, have received special project status.

How might this affect mental health and increased empowerment among those experiencing severe psychological distress? Evidence of structural inequalities exists in relation to mental health as in the case of physical health and ill health. For example, suicide rates show an association with social class and deprivation and both schizophrenia and neurotic states are more commonly diagnosed among people in lower socio-economic groups (for example Meltzer *et al.*, 1995). The White Paper quotes examples of this evidence, including 'children in the poorest households are three times more likely to have mental health problems than children in the best off households' (DoH, 1999, para. 8.4). However, apparently objective evidence about structural inequalities relating to gender and ethnicity and mental health is suspect because of the gendered and racialised definitions used to 'measure' evidence of mental health status. The issue of 'inequality' and mental health is thus perhaps more complex than in the case of, for example, inequality and CHD. However, the legitimation of action to address health inequalities as an increasingly core element of health policy opens up possibilities for strategies which address the disempowerment and exclusion of people experiencing severe psychological distress.

Central to this is the questioning of the adequacy of the medical model to either account for or 'prescribe' appropriate action to improve health status. Once the centrality of medicine is questioned and the need to understand social, economic and environmental factors is accepted, then investment of resources in action to improve the conditions within which distress is experienced is a legitimate part of a health improvement strategy. Hoggett *et al.* (1999) argue that one way of doing this is to reframe mental health in a way which brings it into the mainstream by making the connections between community wellbeing and strategies to cope with depression, anxiety and life crises. This is just the approach adopted by NAG in their public awareness campaigns in Nottingham.

There is also the possibility of action that can enable people to become empowered through improving their economic circumstances and their self-esteem through work opportunities. One example of this is the plans by East London and the City Health Authority to invest in action to improve mental health as part of their HAZ programme. 'Mental illness' is identified as one of the two top causes of ill health, disability and preventable death in the area. Among their proposed plans are initiatives to address the mental health needs of black men and of Asian women, and to develop employment and training opportunities for people who have identified mental health support needs (ELCHA HAZ, 1998). Similarly

Bradford HAZ includes plans to address education, employment and social activities relating to people experiencing severe psychological distress. Bradford's plans go further and, in the context of a work stream on mental health, they also aim to promote community safety, support general community involvement in health to encourage wellbeing, fight poverty and other causes of stress and encourage healthy workplaces free from damaging stress (Bradford HAZ, 1998). The success of such initiatives remains to be seen and the capacity of local initiatives such as these to address many of the structural economic factors which underpin health inequalities is obviously limited. But the objectives of such initiatives are consistent with the broader objective of the users/survivors movement in making the links between the experience of severe psychological distress, stress, poverty and social exclusion.

As well as the substantive content of initiatives which reflect the need to address the root causes of poor health, one of the central characteristics of HAZs is that they are based on notions of partnership – not only between statutory agencies, the voluntary and private sector, but also partnerships with the communities which are the targets of health improvement. Communities in the context of HAZs are understood to include both communities of place and of identity. Thus action is based in localities, in particular those with significant indicators of poor health, and in work with minority ethnic groups, young people, and older people. Community participation in HAZs is intended to contribute directly to health improvement objectives as well as to increase local accountability and improve social cohesion. A variety of mechanisms have been identified through which community representation will be sought on partnership boards or at more local level in determining local action programmes. Community development methods are also being used with a range of different groups as a means of taking direct action to improve health. Community participation in HAZs is seen as a route to empowerment. The objective is for communities to become actively engaged not only in defining the problems as they see them, but also in developing locally appropriate strategies to overcome them. The hypothesis is that engagement provides opportunities for marginalised and excluded communities to have their voices heard and to develop skills and self-esteem that are health enhancing in themselves as well as a means of ensuring greater accountability.

The strategies being developed in at least some areas of the UK in the context of HAZs and other initiatives with health improvement objectives have certain of the characteristics of what Tudor has termed 'Community

Mental Health Promotion' (Tudor, 1996). Tudor considers the potential for functionalist models of mental health promotion (as indeed health promotion generally) to adopt deterministic and static notions of 'good mental health' and to blame individuals for not subscribing to them. In advocating the need for health promoting strategies he suggests that mental health education may comprise information to support strategies for *not* using mental health services. Further he argues that an approach which avoids the deterministic dangers of functionalist approaches needs to include: 'the promotion of social and psychological functioning and development; the promotion of relations and relationships including, for instance, their contradictions; the promotion of the abilities and capacities of individuals, groups and communities; and the promotion of social change in support of mental health' (ibid.: 112).

Early evidence of the experience of community involvement in developing and implementing HAZs indicates the realities of unequal power relationships in attempts to develop partnership approaches (Judge *et al.*, 1999). We are not suggesting that merely announcing a commitment to partnership working, and to addressing the socio-economic factors implicated in poor mental health, will mean that the empowerment objectives of the users/survivors movement are realised. But such developments do represent a shift in the dominant discourse about health in general. In doing so they open up spaces in which initiatives such as Ecoworks (see Chapter 3) or the 'Strategies for Living' project (see Chapter 7) may have more of a chance of securing the resources necessary to sustain their contribution to the development of alternative, more empowering approaches to the experience of psychological distress.

We do, however, also need to identify other aspects of the current climate that may be less favourable to addressing the multiple dimensions of disempowerment discussed in Chapter 1. An appeal to 'community' does not necessarily represent an appeal to inclusivity or tolerance of difference. The more conservative versions of communitarianism are explicitly concerned with conformity to social norms and with individual responsibility for improving one's lot (Etzioni, 1995). There is certainly substantial evidence that public policy, not only for health improvement but across a range of 'cross-cutting policy issues', is considered to require the active contribution of individuals and communities prepared to adjust their own behaviour if policy objectives are to be met (Barnes and Prior, 2000).

A communitarian perspective on the intersecting areas of public health and community safety can lead to some profoundly exclusionary responses to people experiencing severe psychological distress. Etzioni concludes his chapter on 'New Responsibilities: Public Health and Public Safety' with the following:

> even in the most intact communities, some individuals will – because of genetic, chemical, or physiological aberrations or deep-seated psychological distortions – act in an immoral manner. There is a hard core of psychopaths and criminals that the most dedicated parents, the most effective schools, and the most attentive and caring neighbourhoods cannot reach. To cope with them, all communities require the hand of public authorities, lest people be subject to serial killers; wilding gangs out to torture, maim and kill for kicks; child abusers and arsonists. To suggest that these people can be reached by involving them in positive community work, meaningful creative work, or national service is a fairy tale. They are the proper subjects for police. Their legal rights should be fully protected, but otherwise there is no denying that when it comes to hard-core criminals and dangerous mental patients, public authorities are not only essential, but a legitimate, morally appropriate way to protect the public. (Etzioni, op. cit.: 191)

We were writing this just as the Labour Government was announcing proposals that would enable 'untreatable' personality disordered people to be held in secure accommodation when there was an assessed risk that they might commit a violent offence. The easy elision between 'hard-core criminals' and 'dangerous mental patients' continues to feed public perceptions of 'mental illness' as a source of public danger. This is despite evidence that crime is a contributory factor to the experience of severe psychological distress, and that people experiencing such distress are often the victims of aggression and violence. Research in progress indicates that people experiencing severe psychological distress often also experience harassment and intimidation, which goes unreported because people fear they will not be believed or will be considered 'unreliable' witnesses if cases were to come to court (McCabe and Ford, 1999). This and previous research (Wilson and Francis, 1997) has also suggested that black people and openly gay people with mental health problems are uncertain whether they are targeted because of their ethnicity or sexuality, or because of their mental health problems. Whatever the primary source of harassment, the experience is of multiple dimensions of exclusion.

The notion of 'community justice' (Nellis, 1999) is perhaps more consistent than that of community safety with the aspirations of users/survivors movements seeking the empowerment of people who have often been excluded from community as a result of the fear of the otherness represented by madness. An appeal to 'justice' might raise questions about legislating powers to exercise preventive control only in cases where there is an assessment of future risk based on the mental state of the individual concerned. One argument which is put concerns why such powers are not being proposed in other cases where the risk assessment may be more certain – in the case of people known to create violent disturbance at football matches, for example.

So what are the prospects for increasing the empowerment of people in relation to those services designed specifically for people experiencing severe psychological distress?

Enabling participation

In the light of the evidence, that we have discussed in Chapters 5 and 6, of the potential for empowerment strategies to both assist individuals experiencing distress and to enhance the value of the services that are offered to them, we would like to be optimistic about the possibilities for further development of that impact. We have, in particular, stressed the critical role that professionals can play by their attitudes and actions in encouraging action and providing practical support to users striving to empower themselves.

We think that if empowerment strategies are to have an impact, professionals working directly with service users need to change. One central need is for a greater shared understanding of what is expected to be gained from user involvement. Individuals who are drawn in or cajoled into participation in particular committees or groups are often uncertain about what is expected of them or what they can be expected to achieve. If they find they are not able to make the contribution expected or achieve what they have set out to achieve, this can lead to disillusionment and a reluctance to participate subsequently – it can be a disempowering experience. Many of those participating in user committees within institutions are particularly unclear about their purpose and cynical about their effectiveness. Partly this reflects a view still held by some professionals that the central purpose of participation is a therapeutic one rather than to give service users a route to influence the services intended to alleviate their distress. What is needed here is a clear understanding on the part of professionals of what goals service users set for participation and some negotiation about what powers and responsibilities might therefore be usefully devolved to user committees. Adopting such an approach and regularly reviewing the purpose and form of such participation with service users – setting up a dynamic relationship over which service users have some power and influence – is probably more important in promoting empowerment than prescribing involvement in particular activities such as staff selection or particular management activities.

Broader decision-making within service organisations

We have also identified similar differences, between service users and those responsible for broader decision-making within service organisations, in the goals of user involvement in that decision-making. Nor is it always clear that organisations are drawing in service users rather than their carers or sympathetic supporters from voluntary organisations, nor indeed that these distinctions are always clearly made. Furthermore, there remain concerns from policy-makers about the representativeness of service users, in particular the idea that articulate interested service users might not reflect the views of the 'typical' user. Nor is there always a recognition that service users are not homogenous groups – that, for example, black service users might have particular needs and views or that women might have a different perspective than men. This can be reflected by apprehension on the part of service users about their role and has led to some user representatives withdrawing, particularly where they identify pressure to justify their position.

Partly this reflects the different goals of policy makers, concerned about the legitimacy of the processes of making decisions about the services they offer and a desire to gain as representative a view as they can about what services are appropriate for the majority of those they serve, and of individual service user groups who quite properly are pursuing the particular interests of those who make up their active membership. Further dissonance may be created by the pursuit by service user groups of goals that go further than the remit of particular service organisations or the purposes of particular consultation exercises, as was shown so starkly in the Canadian context by the problems highlighted by Church (1996). It is critical in this respect that service organisations develop a greater understanding of the goals and forms of organisation of the users/survivors movement rather than expecting it to fit neatly into their expectations. We have shown how working relationships can be established in the particular context of the Purchasing for Users Group in Nottingham and the Mental Health Services Users Group in Newcastle.

It would be wrong to imply, however, that the facilitation of more meaningful dialogue simply requires changes in the individual attitudes of professionals or policy makers. It should not be forgotten that existing decision-making structures are designed around the expectations of those traditionally involved – confident, experienced local politicians and full-time professionals. These service users may share experiences and attributes – and some do. User groups like NAG have also undertaken development programmes designed to equip members for exactly such participation. However, if organisations are serious about incorporating the unique experience of service users, they need to consider the very format of their relationships with the users/survivors movement. This means undertaking exercises particularly designed to facilitate that participation, such as that described by Pilgrim and Waldron (1998), and taking risks in their relationships with service user organisations by entering into genuine negotiation about what the goals and format of such participation might be – reflecting a commitment to a more equal partnership.

Training and education

Training may have a critical role to play. Many organisations' mission statements now include reference to a commitment to user participation. Entry to post-qualifying social work courses is only open to those demonstrating an understanding of user perspectives and a commitment to user empowerment. Yet our own research and other research reviewed here has shown that both service users themselves and fellow professionals identify a reluctance on the part of those working within the system to alter cherished ways of working as a major barrier to change. Even where there is genuine sympathy for user empowerment, the research has identified the gulf between service users and those working within the system in their understanding of what that empowerment really implies. There is an urgent need to develop policy-maker and professional understanding of the rich variety of organisational forms and objectives of the users/survivors movement if meaningful dialogue is to be extended. Mental health professionals also need to be given the opportunity to develop an understanding that the development of user input into decision making, while implying changes in their practice, is not simply about losing power to another group. Indeed, if it results in policies and working practices that are based on an enriched and more authentic knowledge base, it will enhance their 'power to'. This will not be achieved by organisations that are developing empowerment strategies simply running short joint training courses for both users and staff, where they are exposed to each others' perspectives, doubts and fears. Indeed, useful though these are, both service users and professional staff also need separate opportunities to work through these anxieties, and develop their expectations of user empowerment and its implications for them, if those joint activities are going to be of benefit. Nor should an occasional day or module on 'user perspectives' be seen as sufficient service user input into basic or post-qualifying training.

Our hope is to see an extension of the examples we identified in Chapter 3 of partnership in training – where service users have taken on roles as core trainers and advisors on training and educational development. This will enable them to bring to courses reflections, based on their own experience as well as information about the commitments and desires of the user movement, into consideration of every aspect of the knowledge base of mental health professionals. It is only with that degree of involvement that we are likely to see a genuine shift in the paradigm within which mental health professionals are trained, in which the experiential knowledge of users has a recognised central place.

Involvement strategies and movement goals

We ourselves have been among those advocating the development of more holistic user empowerment strategies within service agencies (Bowl, 1996b). We continue to believe that organisations, which are genuinely committed to changing their practice to encompass greater influence for service users on services delivered and how they are shaped, need to develop such comprehensive strategies. These must include: consideration of the appropriateness of different forms of decision making and the impact of traditional structures on relative newcomers to the process; consideration of how to support service users in overcoming the legacy of powerlessness, often engendered by that role, so that they feel able to exercise their own expert status within decision-making and development processes; show understanding of and avoid the negative implications of specifically questioning service users 'representativeness' while confronting the need to facilitate representation of diversity within service user populations; and efforts to overcome the barriers to staff acceptance of the legitimacy of service user participation.

However important such efforts might be, it would, nonetheless, be wrong in our view to assume that the major influence on the developing nature of the relationships between UK mental health services and their users will come from the actions of service providers. The key factor will surely be how the mental health service user movement itself develops. The extent to which its pursuit of the goals we have outlined in Chapters 3 and 7 continues to bring it into contact with existing service providers may well change. We may see, as has happened in the USA, further development of separation from those services and the development of alternative service user controlled provision. We may see, as further opportunities open up for the sorts of partnership discussed earlier in this chapter, a switch in goals, away from concern to influence remedial services to a greater focus on what service users have identified as their primary concerns – employment, housing and social networks. Developments in service user movement activity may also change the pattern of interaction with existing service providers in another way – as service user achievements further challenge the perceptions, built into the knowledge base of professionals, of the limitations to service user autonomy. In other words service users and professionals are engaged in a dynamic interactive process, the outcome of which we cannot predict.

What we already see as a positive development, within mental health services, is a much more rounded and complex understanding of the process and nature of 'empowerment' than was offered by the consumerist discourse of the 1980s and early 1990s. Whatever the limitations of the official rhetoric of 'partnership', this is a more useful starting point for the development of empowerment strategies than that offered by an appeal to 'consumer choice'. Partnership has the capacity to offer something of value to both user and provider of services by placing greater responsibilities on both to engage in a new type of relationship. Such a relationship, that harnesses the knowledge and experience of each, can create better individual outcomes. It can also construct new understandings of the origins and nature of the experience of psychological distress in the context of community life, which may itself need to be a focus for strategies that contribute to mental health and empowerment.

References

Acheson, D. (1998) *Independent Inquiry into Inequalities in Health.* London, HMSO.

Afshar, H. (ed.) (1998) *Women and Empowerment. Illustrations from the Third World.* Basingstoke, Macmillan.

Albany Videos (1986) *We're Not Mad... We're Angry.* London, Albany Videos.

Allen, H. (1987) *Justice Unbalanced. Gender: Psychiatry and Judicial Decisions.* Milton Keynes, Open University Press.

Altman, D. (1994) *Power and Community. Organizational and Cultural Responses to AIDS.* London, Taylor and Francis.

Anderson, J. (1996) 'Yes, but IS IT Empowerment? Initiation, Implementation and Outcomes of Community Action', in Humphries, B (ed.) *Critical Perspectives on Empowerment.* Birmingham, Venture Press.

Anderson, J. M. (1996) 'Empowering Patients: Issues and Strategies', *Social Science and Medicine,* **43**(5): 697–705.

Angstringen-Oslo (1995) *Summary of an Evaluation Survey Carried out among Participants in Angstringen-Oslo's Self-organised Self-help Groups.* Angstringen-Oslo, Norway.

Ashton, H. (1991) 'Psychotropic Drug Prescribing for Women', *British Journal of Psychiatry,* **158**: 30–5.

Atkin, K. (1991) 'Community Care in a Multi-racial Society: Incorporating the User View', *Policy and Politics,* **19**(3): 159–66.

Bailey, D. (1997) 'What is the Way Forward for a User-led Approach to the Delivery of Mental Health Services in Primary Care?', *Journal of Mental Health,* **6**(1): 101–5.

Baker, P. (1997) 'From Victims to Allies: A Practical Way Forward in Forging Alliances', *Nursing Times,* **93**(27): 42.

Banton, R., Clifford, P., Frosh, S., Lousada, J. and Rosenthall, J. (1985) *The Politics of Mental Health.* Basingstoke, Macmillan.

Barham, P. (1992) *Closing the Asylum. The Mental Patient in Modern Society.* Harmondsworth, Penguin.

Barker, I. and Peck, E. (1987) *Power in Strange Places. User Empowerment in Mental Health Services.* London, Good Practices in Mental Health.

Barnes, C. and Mercer, G. (eds) (1997) *Doing Disability Research.* Leeds, Disability Press.

Barnes, M. (1996) 'Challenging the Culture: Representing the Rights of Women in Special Hospitals', in Hemingway, C. (ed.) *Special Women? The Experience of Women in the Special Hospital System.* Aldershot, Avebury.

Barnes, M. (1997a) *Care, Communities and Citizens.* Harlow, Addison Wesley Longman.

Barnes, M. (1997b) *The People's Health Service?* Birmingham, The NHS Confederation.

Barnes, M. (1997c) 'Families and Empowerment', in P. Ramcharan *et al.* (eds) *Empowerment in Everyday Life: Learning Disability.* London, Jessica Kingsley.

Barnes, M. (1999a) *Building a Deliberative Democracy: An Evaluation of Two Citizens' Juries.* London, IPPR.

Barnes, M. (1999b) 'Public Expectations. From Paternalism to Partnership: Changing Relationships in Health and Health Services' No.10 in the Technical Series: *Policy Futures for UK Health.* London, Nuffield Trust.

Barnes, M. (1999c) 'Users as Citizens: Collective Action and the Local Governance of Welfare', *Social Policy and Administration,* **33**(1): 73–90.

Barnes, M. and Maple, N. (1992) *Women and Mental Health: Challenging the Stereotypes.* Birmingham, Venture Press.

Barnes, M. and Prior, D. (1995) 'Spoilt for Choice? How Consumerism can Disempower Public Service Users', *Public Money and Management,* **15**(3): 53–8.

Barnes, M. and Prior, D. (2000) *Private Lives as Public Policy,* Imagining Welfare Futures Series. Birmingham, Venture Press.

Barnes, M. and Shardlow, P. (1996) 'Identity Crisis? Mental Health User Groups and the "Problem" of Identity', in Barnes, C. and Mercer, G. (eds) *Exploring the Divide: Illness and Disability.* Leeds, Disability Press.

Barnes, M. and Shardlow, P. (1997) 'From Passive Recipient to Active Citizen: Participation in Mental Health User Groups', *Journal of Mental Health,* **6**(3): 289–300.

Barnes, M. and Stephenson, P. (1996) 'Secure Provision – The Special Hospitals', in Perkins *et al.* (ibid.) p. 176).

Barnes, M. and Walker, A. (1996) 'Consumerism versus Empowerment: A Principled Approach to the Involvement of Older Service Users', *Policy and Politics,* **24**(4): 375–93.

Barnes, M. and Warren, L. (eds) (1999) *Paths to Empowerment.* Bristol, Policy Press.

Barnes, M. and Wistow, G. (1994a) 'Achieving a Strategy for User Involvement in Community Care', *Health and Social Care in the Community,* **2**: 347–56.

Barnes, M. and Wistow, G. (1994b) 'Learning to Hear Voices: Listening to Users of Mental Health Services', *Journal of Mental Health,* **3**: 525–40.

Barnes, M., Bowl, R. and Fisher, M. (1990) *Sectioned: Social Services and the 1983 Mental Health Act.* London, Routledge.

Barnes, M., Harrison, S., Mort, M. and Shardlow, P. (1999a) *Unequal Partners – User Groups and Community Care.* Bristol, Policy Press.

Barnes, M., Harrison, S., Mort, M., Shardlow, P. and Wistow, G. (1996) *Consumerism and Citizenship amongst users of Health and Social Care Services.* Final report to ESRC of Award No. L311253025.

Barnes, M., Harrison, S., Mort, M., Shardlow, P. and Wistow, G. (1999b) 'The New Management of Community Care: User Groups, Citizenship and Co-production', in Stoker, G. (ed.) *The New Management of British Local Governance.* Basingstoke and New York, Macmillan.

Barton, L. (1993) 'The Struggle for Citizenship: The Case of Disabled People', *Disability, Handicap and Society,* **8**(3): 235–48.

Batsleer, J (1999) 'Rethinking Citizenship: Questions of Voice and Dialogue in Welfare Practice'. Paper given to the Rethinking Citizenship Conference, Leeds University, June.

Bean, P., Bingley, W., Bynoe, I. *et al.* (1991) *Out of Harm's Way*. London, MIND.

Beliappa, J. (1991) *Illness or Distress? Alternative Models of Mental Health*. London, Confederation of Indian Organisations.

Beresford, P. and Croft, S. (1986) *Whose Welfare: Private Care or Public Services?* Brighton, Lewis Cohen Urban Studies Centre.

Bernlef, J. (1988) *Out of Mind*. London, Faber and Faber.

Blumer, H. (1995) 'Social Movements', in Lyman, S. (ed.) *Social Movements: Critiques, Concepts, Case Studies*. Basingstoke, Macmillan.

Bock, G. and James, S. (eds) (1992) *Beyond Equality and Difference*. London, Routledge.

Bolton, P. (1984) 'Management of Compulsory Admitted Patients to a High Security Unit', *International Journal of Social Psychiatry*, **30**: 77–84.

Bond, J., Newnes, C. and Mooniaruch, F. (1992) 'User Views of the Inpatient Psychiatric Service at Shelton Hospital', *Clinical Psychology Forum*, **49**: 21–6.

Boushel, M. and Farmer, E. (1996) 'Work with Families where Children are at Risk: Control and/or Empowerment?', in Parslow, P. (ed.) *Pathways to Empowerment*. Birmingham, Venture Press.

Bowl, R. (1996a) 'Involving Service Users in Mental Health Services: Social Services Departments and the National Health Service and Community Care Act 1990', *Journal of Mental Health*, **5**(3): 287–303.

Bowl, R. (1996b) 'Legislating for User Involvement in the United Kingdom; Mental Health Services and the NHS and Community Care Act 1990', *International Journal of Social Psychiatry*, **42**(3): 165–80.

Bowl, R. and Barnes, M. (1993) 'Approved Social Worker Assessments, Race and Racism', in Clarke, P., Harrison, M., Patel, K., Shah, M., Varley, M. and Zack-Williams, T. (eds) *Improving Mental Health Practice*. London, CCETSW.

Bowl, R. and Ross, K. (1994) *Training for Democracy: Involving Users in Adult Services*, Monograph 1. University of Birmingham School of Continuing Studies.

Bradford Health Action Zone (1998) *Breaking Barriers – Improving Health. Practical Steps to Better Health*. Bradford Health Authority/Bradford Metropolitan District Council.

Brandon, D. (1991) *Innovation Without Change?* Basingstoke, Macmillan.

Brandon, D. (1992) Opening Speech, *Skills for People Annual Report and National Conference Report*. Newcastle Upon Tyne, Skills for People.

Braye, S. and Preston-Shoot, M. (1995) *Empowering Practice in Social Care*. Buckingham, Open University Press.

Briere, J. and Zaidi, L.V. (1989) 'Sexual Abuse Histories and Sequelae in Female Psychiatric Emergency Room Patients', *American Journal of Psychiatry*, **12**: 1601–6.

Brown, G. and Harris, T. (1978) *Social Origins of Depression: A Study of Psychiatric Disorder in Women*. London, Tavistock.

Brown, G.R. and Anderson, B. (1991) 'Psychiatric Morbidity in Adult Inpatients with Childhood Histories of Sexual and Physical Abuse', *American Journal of Psychiatry*, **148**: 55–61.

Browne, D. (1990) *Black People, Mental Health and the Courts*. London, NACRO.

Browne, D. (1996) 'The Black Experience of Mental Health Law', Ch. 23 in Heller, T. *et al.* (eds) *Mental Health Matters*. London, Macmillan.

Bryer, J.B., Nielson, B.A., Miller, J.B. and Krol, P.A. (1987) 'Childhood Sexual Abuse and Physical Abuse as Factors in Adult Psychiatric Illness', *American Journal of Psychiatry*, **144**(1): 1426–31.

Busfield, J. (1986) *Managing Madness*. London, Unwin Hyman.

Busfield, J. (1996) *Men, Women and Madness. Understanding Gender and Mental Disorder*. Basingstoke, Macmillan.

Campbell, B. (1988) *Unofficial Secrets. Child Sexual Abuse: The Cleveland Case*. London, Virago.

Campbell, J. and Oliver, M. (1996) *Disability Politics. Understanding our Past, Changing our Future*. London, Routledge.

Caron, J. and Bergeron, N. (1995) 'A Self-help Partnership Group for People who have Experienced Psychiatric Hospitalization: An Exploratory Study'. *Canada's Mental Health*, **43**(2): 19–28.

Carpenter, J. and Sbaraini, S. (1996) 'Involving Service Users and Carers in the Care Programme Approach', *Journal of Mental Health*, **5**(5): 483–8.

Chamberlin, J. (1988) *On Our Own*. London, MIND.

Chen, E., Harrison, G. and Standen, P. (1991) 'Management of First Episode Psychotic Illness in Afro-Caribbean Patients', *British Journal of Psychiatry*, **158**: 517–22.

Church, K. (1996) 'Beyond "Bad Manners": The Power Relations of "Consumer Participation" in Ontario's Community Mental Health System', *Canadian Journal of Community Mental Health*, **15**(2): 27–44.

Church, K. and Reville, D. (1989) 'User Involvement in the Mental Health Field in Canada', *Canada's Mental Health*, **37**: 22–5.

Clayton, S. (1988) 'Patient Participation : An Undeveloped Concept', *Journal of the Royal Society of Health*, **108**(2): 55–6, 58.

Cochrane, R. (1983) *The Social Creation of Mental Illness*. London, Longman.

Cochrane, R. and Bal, S.S. (1989) 'Mental Hospital Admission Rates of Immigrants to England: A Comparison of 1971 and 1981', *Social Psychiatry and Psychiatric Epidemiology*, **24**: 2–11.

Coe, A. (1992) The Consumer Movement and Mental Health Service Users. Unpublished MSoc.Sci. Dissertation, University of Birmingham, Department of Social Policy and Social Work.

Cohen, J.L. (1985) 'Strategy or Identity: New Theoretical Paradigms and Contemporary Social Movements', *Social Research*, **52**(4): 663–716.

Cope, R. (1989) 'The Compulsory Detention of Afro-Caribbeans under the Mental Health Act', *New Community*, **15**(3): 343–56.

Corbett, J. (1994) 'A Proud Label: Exploring the Relationship between Disability Politics and Gay Pride', *Disability and Society*, **9**(3): 343–57.

Croft, S. and Beresford, P. (1990) *From Paternalism to Participation: Involving People in Social Services*. London, Open Services Project/Joseph Rowntree Foundation.

Crossley, N. (1998) 'Transforming the Mental Health Field: The Early History of the National Association for Mental Health', *Sociology of Health and Illness*, **20**(4): 458–88.

Curran, T. (1997) 'Power, Participation and Post Modernism: User and Practitioner Participation in Mental Health Social Work Education,' *Social Work Education*, **16**(3): 21–36.

Curran, V. and Golombok, S. (1985) *Bottling It Up*. London, Faber and Faber.

Dalton, R.J., Kuechler, M. and Burklin, W. (1990) 'The Challenge of New Movements', in Dalton, R.J. and Kuechler, M. (eds) *Challenging the Political Order. New Social and Political Movements in Western Democracies*. Cambridge, Polity Press.

Davey, B. (1994) 'Mental Health and the Environment', *Care in Place*, **1**(2): 188–210.

Davey, B. (1999) 'Solving Economic, Social and Environmental Problems Together: An Empowerment Strategy for Losers', in Barnes, M. and Warren, L. (eds) *Alliances and Partnerships in Empowerment*. Bristol, Policy Press.

Davis, A. (1981) *Women, Race and Class*. New York, Random House.

Davis, A. and Betteridge, J. (1997) *Mental Health and Welfare to Work*. London, Mental Health Foundation.

Davis, L.J. (1995) *Enforcing Normalcy: Disability, Deafness and the Body*. London, Verso.

DoH (Department of Health) (1989) *Caring for People: Community Care into the Next Decade and Beyond*. White Paper, Cmd. 849, London, HMSO.

DoH (Department of Health) (1990) *Caring for People Implementation Documents. Draft Guidance: Planning*. London, DoH.

DoH (Department of Health) (1992) *The Health of the Nation*. London, HMSO.

DoH (Department of Health) (1993) *Changing Childbirth. Part 2: Survey of Good Communications Practice in Maternity Services*. London, HMSO.

DoH (Department of Health) (1994) *Working in Partnership*. London, HMSO.

DoH (Department of Health) (1995) *Building Bridges*. London, HMSO.

DoH (Department of Health) (1998) *Modernising Mental Health Services. Safe, Sound and Supportive*. London, DoH.

DoH (Department of Health) (1999) *Saving Lives: Our Healthier Nation*, Cm 4386. London, HMSO.

Dominelli, L. (1990) *Women and Community Action*. Birmingham, Venture Press.

Doyal, L. (1995) *What Makes Women Sick. Gender and the Political Economy of Health*. Basingstoke, Macmillan.

Doyal, L. and Gough, I. (1991) *A Theory of Human Need*. Basingstoke, Macmillan.

Ehrenreich, B. and English, D. (1979) *For Her Own Good. 150 Years of the Experts' Advice to Women*. London, Pluto Press.

ELCHA Health Action Zone (1998) *Breaking the Cycle*. East London and the City Health Authority.

Ellis, K. (1993) *Squaring the Circle. User and Carer Participation in Needs Assessment*. York, Joseph Rowntree Foundation.

Ernst, S. and Maguire, M. (eds) (1987) *Living with the Sphinx*. London, Women's Press.

Etzioni, A. (1995) *The Spirit of Community. Rights, Responsibilities and the Communitarian Agenda*. London, Fontana.

Everett, B. (1994) 'Something is Happening: The Contemporary Consumer and Psychiatric Survivor Movement in Historical Context', *Journal of Mind and Behavior*, **15**(1–2): 55–70.

Everett, B. (1998) 'Participation or Exploitation? Consumers and Psychiatric Survivors as Partners in Planning Mental Health Services', *International Journal of Mental Health*, **27**(1): 80–97.

Faulkner, A. (1997) *Knowing our Own Minds*. London, Mental Health Foundation.

Fennell, M. (1977) 'Learned Helplessness in the Aged: A Study of Two Local Authority Old People's Homes'. MSc. Dissertation, University of Birmingham, Department of Psychology.

Fenton, S. and Sadiq-Sangster, A. (1996) 'Culture, Relativism and the Expression of Mental Distress: South Asian Women in Britain', *Sociology of Health and Illness*, **18**(1): 66–85.

Fernando, S. (1991) *Mental Health Race and Culture*. London, Macmillan.

Fetterman, D.M., Kaftarian, S.J. and Wandersman, A. (eds) (1996) *Empowerment Evaluation. Knowledge and Tools for Self-assessment and Accountability*. Thousand Oaks, CA, Sage.

Figert, A. (1996) *Women and the Ownership of PMS. The Structuring of a Psychiatric Disorder*. New York, Aldine de Gruyter.

Flynn, N. (1993) *Public Sector Management*. Hemel Hempstead, Harvester Wheatsheaf.

Forbes, J. and Sashidharan, S.P. (1997) 'User Involvement in Services – Incorporation or Challenge?', *British Journal of Social Work*, **27**(4): 481–98.

Foucault, M. (1965) *Madness and Civilization. A History of Insanity in the Age of Reason*. London, Tavistock.

Foucault, M. (1980) *Power/Knowledge, Selected Interviews and Other Writings, 1972–1977*. Edited by Colin Gordon, Brighton, Harvester.

Fraser, S. (1989) *My Father's House. A Memoir of Incest and of Healing*. London, Virago.

Frederick, J. (1991) *Positive Thinking for Mental Health*. London, Black Mental Health Group.

French, S. (1993) 'Disability, Impairment or Something in Between?', in Swain, J., Finkelstein, V., French, S. and Oliver, M. (eds) *Disabling Barriers – Enabling Environments*. London, Sage.

Gaster, L., Harrison, L., Martin, L., Means, R. and Thistlethwaite, P. (eds) (1993) *Working Together for Better Community Care*. Bristol, School for Advanced Urban Studies, University of Bristol.

Gell, C. (1987) 'Learning to Lobby. The Growth of Patients' Council in Nottingham', in Barker, I. and Peck, E. (eds) *Power in Strange Places. User Empowerment in Mental Health Services*. London, Good Practices in Mental Health.

Giddens, A. (1998) *The Third Way*. Cambridge, Polity Press.

Gilroy, P. (1987) *There Ain't No Black in the Union Jack*. London, Hutchinson.

Glendinning, C. and Bewley, C. (1992) *Involving Disabled People in Community Care Planning – The First Steps*. Manchester, Department of Social Policy and Social Work, University of Manchester.

Goffman, E. (1968) *Asylums – Essays on the Social Situation of Mental Patients and Other Inmates*. London, Penguin.

Good Practices in Mental Health (1994) 'Women and Mental Health'. An information pack of mental health services for women in the United Kingdom. Produced by Good Practices in Mental Health in collaboration with the European Regional Council, World Federation for Mental Health, London.

Gordon, R.E. *et al.* (1982) 'Reducing Hospitalization of State Mental Patients: Peer Management and Support', in Yaeger, A. and Slotkin, R. (eds) *Community Mental Health*. New York, Plenum.

Gostin, L., Meacher, M. and Olsen, M.R. (1983) *The 1983 Mental Health Act: A Guide for Social Workers*. Birmingham, British Association of Social Workers.

Greenberg, J., Greenley, J.R. and Benedict, P. (1994) 'Contributions of People with Serious Mental Illness to their Families', *Hospital and Community Psychiatry*, **45**: 475–80.

Gutierrez, L.M., DeLois, K.A. and GlenMaye, L. (1995) 'Understanding Empowerment Practice: Building on Practitioner-based Knowledge', *Families in Society*, **7**(9): 534–42.

Gyford, J. (1991) *Citizens, Consumers and Councils. Local Government and the Public*. Basingstoke, Macmillan.

Habermas, J. (1981) 'New Social Movements', *Telos*, **48**: 33–7.

Hancock, T. (1993) 'The Healthy City from Conception to Application: Implications for Research', in Davies, J.K. and Kelly, M.P. (eds) *Healthy Cities: Research and Practice*. London, Routledge.

Hannigan, B., Bartlett, H. and Clilverd, A. (1997) 'Improving Health and Social Functioning: Perspectives of Mental Health Service Users', *Journal of Mental Health*, **6**(6): 613–19.

Harding, S. (1991) *Whose Science. Whose Knowledge? Thinking from Women's Lives*. Milton Keynes, Open University Press.

Harrison, G., Owens, D., Holton, A., Neilson, D. and Boot, D. (1988) 'A Prospective Study of Severe Mental Disorder in Afro-Caribbean Patients', *Psychological Medicine*, **18**: 643–57.

Harrison, G., Holton, A., Neilson, D., Owens, D., Boot, D. and Cooper, J. (1989) 'Severe Mental Disorder in Afro-Caribbean Patients: Some Social, Demographic and Service Factors', *Psychological Medicine*, **19**: 683–96.

Harrison, L. (1993) 'Newcastle's Mental Health Services Consumer Group. A Case Study of User Involvement', in Gaster, L., Harrison, L., Martin, L., Means, R. and Thistlethwaite, P. (eds) *Working Together for Better Community Care*. Bristol, School for Advanced Urban Studies, University of Bristol.

Hart, L. (1995) *Phone At Nine Just To Say You're Alive*. Lutterworth, Abbott Press.

Hepplewhite, R. (1988) 'Introduction' in Common Concerns. International Conference on User Involvement in Mental Health Services. University of Sussex, Brighton: East Sussex County Council, Brighton Health Authority, MIND.

Hewitt, M. (1993) 'Social Movements and Social Need: Problems with Postmodern Political Theory', *Critical Social Policy*, **37**, Summer: 52–74.

Higgins, R. (1993) 'Evaluation of the Richmond Fellowship Advocacy Project, Wakefield', Project paper 2, University of Leeds, Nuffield Institute for Health.

Hoggett, P., Stewart, M., Razzaque, K. and Barker, I. (1999) *Urban Regeneration and Mental Health in London*. London, King's Fund.

Hogman, G. and Chapman, M. (1998) *Surviving in the Community, NSF Benefits Survey*. Kingston-upon-Thames, National Schizophrenia Fellowship.

Hopton, J. (1995) 'User Involvement in the Education of Mental Health Nurses. An Evaluation of Possibilities', *Critical Social Policy*, **42**: 47–60.

Hoyes, L., Jeffers, S., Lart, R., Means, R. and Taylor, M. (1993) *User Empowerment and the Reform of Community Care: An Interim Assessment*. Bristol, School for Advanced Urban Studies.

Jadhav, S. (1996) 'The Cultural Origins of Western Depression', *International Journal of Social Psychiatry*, **42**(4): 269–86.

James, S. (1992) 'The Good-enough Citizen: Citizenship and Independence', in Bock, G. and James, S. (eds) *Beyond Equality and Difference. Feminist Politics, Female Subjectivity.* London, Routledge.

Jenkins, J.C. (1983) 'Resource Mobilization Theory and the Study of Social Movements', *Annual Review of Sociology*, **9**: 527–53.

Jenkins, J.C. (1987) 'Nonprofit Organizations and Policy Advocacy', in Powell, W.W. (ed.) *The Nonprofit Sector: A Research Handbook.* New Haven, Yale University Press.

Jenkins, R. (1985) 'Sex Differences in Minor Psychiatric Morbidity: A Survey of a Homogeneous Population', *Social Science and Medicine,* **20**(9): 887–99.

Jenner, A. (1988) 'A Psychiatrist's Apologia', in *Common Concerns. International Conference on User Involvement in Mental Health Services.* University of Sussex, Brighton: East Sussex County Council, Brighton Health Authority, MIND.

Jennings, A. (1998) 'On Being Invisible in the Mental Health System', in Levin, B.L., Blanch, A.K. and Jennings, A. (eds) *Women's Mental Health Services: A Public Health Perspective.* Thousand Oaks, CA, Sage.

Jensen, T.O. and Froestad, J. (1988) 'Interest organizations – A Complex Answer to Political Poverty', *Tidscrift for Rattssociolgi,* **5**(2): 85–117.

Jones, G. and Berry, M. (1986) 'Regional Secure Units: The Emerging Picture', in Edwards, G. (ed.) *Current Issues in Clinical Psychology,* 4. London, Plenum Press.

Jones, L. and Lodge, A. (1991) 'A Survey of Psychiatric Patients' Views of Outpatient Clinic Facilities', *Health Bulletin*, **49**: 320–8.

Judge, K., Barnes, M., Bauld, L., Benzeval, M., Killoran, A., Robinson, R., Wigglesworth, R. and Zeilig, H. (1999) *Health Action Zones: Learning to Make a Difference.* Findings from a preliminary review of Health Action Zones and proposals for a national evaluation. Submitted to the Department of Health.

Kalinowski, C. and Penney, D. (1998) 'Empowerment and Women's Mental Health Services', in Lubotsky Levin, B., Blanch, A.K. and Jennings, A. (eds) *Women's Mental Health Services. A Public Health Perspective.* Thousand Oaks, CA, Sage.

Kent, H. and Read, J. (1998) 'Measuring Consumer Participation in Mental Health Services: Are Attitudes Related to Professional Orientation?', *International Journal of Social Psychiatry*, **44**(4): 295–310.

Killick, J. (1998) 'Confidences', *Openmind,* **90**, (March/April): 14–15.

King, M., Coker, E., Leavey, G., Hoare, A. and Johnson-Sabine, E. (1994) 'Incident of Psychotic Illness in London: Comparison of Ethnic Groups', *British Medical Journal,* **309**: 1115–19.

Kleinman, A. (1987) 'Anthropology and Psychiatry: The Role of Culture in Cross-cultural Research on Illness', *British Journal of Psychiatry*, **151**: 447–54.

Kramer, S. and Roberts, J. (eds) 1996) *The Politics of Attachment. Towards a Secure Society.* London, Free Association Books.

Krause, I. (1989) 'Sinking Heart: A Punjabi Communication of Distress', *Social Science and Medicine,* **29**(4): 563–75.

Kriesi, H., Koopmans, R., Dyvendak, J.W. and Giugni, M.G. (1995) *New Social Movements in Western Europe*. London, UCL Press.

Kurtz, L.F. and Chambon, A. (1987) 'Comparison of Self-help Groups for Mental Health', *Health and Social Work*, **12**: 275–83.

Law Commission (1995) *Mental Incapacity, Item 9 of the Fourth Programme of Law Reform: Mentally Incapacitated Adults*. London, HMSO.

Leff, J. (ed.) (1997) *Care in the Community. Illusion or Reality?* Chichester, John Wiley.

Leff, J. and Vaughan, C. (1985) *Expressed Emotion in Families*. New York, Guilford.

Lefley, H.P. (1996) *Family Caregiving in Mental Illness*. Thousand Oaks, CA, Sage.

Lindow, V. (1994) *Self-help Alternatives to Mental Health Services*. London, MIND.

Lindow, V. and Morris, J. (1995) *Service User Involvement. Synthesis of Findings and Experience in the Field of Community Care*. York, Joseph Rowntree Foundation.

Lister, R (1997) *Citizenship. Feminist Perspectives*. Basingstoke, Macmillan.

Littlewood, R. (1992) 'Psychiatric Diagnosis and Racial Bias: Empirical and Interpretative Approaches', *Social Science and Medicine*, **34**(2): 141–9.

Littlewood, R. and Cross, S. (1980) 'Ethnic Minorities and Psychiatric Services', *Sociology of Health and Illness*, **2**: 194–201.

Lord, J. (1989) 'The Potential of Consumer Participation: Sources of Understanding', *Canada's Mental Health*, **37**: 15–17.

Lord, J. and Dufort, F. (1996) 'Power and Oppression in Mental Health', *Canadian Journal of Community Mental Health*, **15**(2): 5–11.

Lord, J., Ochocka, J., Czarny, W. and MacGillivary, H. (1998) 'Analysis of Change Within a Mental Health Organization: A Participatory Process', *Psychiatric Rehabilitation Journal*, **21**(4): 327–39.

Lovenduski, J. and Randall, V. (1993) *Contemporary Feminist Politics. Women and Power in Britain*. Oxford, Oxford University Press.

Lunt, N. and Thornton, P. (1996) 'Disabled People, Work and Benefits. A Review of the Research Literature'. Paper prepared for a Joseph Rowntree Foundation Seminar.

Marsh, P. and Fisher, M. (1992) *Good Intentions: Developing Partnership in Social Services*. York, Joseph Rowntree Foundation.

Marshall, T.H. (1950) *Citizenship and Social Class and Other Essays*. Cambridge, Cambridge University Press.

McCabe, A. and Ford, C. (1999) *Redressing the Balance*. Birmingham, Public Health Alliance.

McCabe, S. and Unzicker, R.E. (1995) 'Changing Roles of Consumer/Survivors in Mature Mental Health Systems', in Stein, L.I., Hollingsworth, E.J. *et al.* (eds) *Maturing Mental Health Systems: New Challenges and Opportunities*. New Directions for Mental Health Services, No 66, San Francisco, Jossey-Bass.

McGovern, D. and Cope, R. (1987) 'First Psychiatric Admission Rates of First and Second Generation Afro-Caribbeans', *Social Psychiatry*, **22**: 139–49.

McGrath, M. (1989) 'Consumer Participation in Service Planning – the AWS Experience', *Journal of Social Policy*, **18**(1): 67–89.

McKenzie, K., van Os, J., Fahy, T., Jones, P., Harvey, I., Toone, B. and Murray, R. (1995) 'Psychosis with Good Prognosis in Afro-Caribbean People now Living in the United Kingdom', *British Medical Journal*, **311**: 1325–8.

McLean, A. (1995) 'Empowerment and the Psychiatric Consumer/Ex-patient Movement in the United States: Contradictions, Crisis and Change', *Social Science and Medicine*, **40**(8): 1053–107.

McMurphy's (1996) *McMurphy's Users Review... 1996*. Sheffield, McMurphy's.

Meltzer, H., Gill, B., Petticrew, M. and Hinds, K. (1995) *The Prevalence of Psychiatric Morbidity Among Adults Living in Private Households, OPCS Surveys of Psychiatric Morbidity in Great Britain, Report 1*. London, HMSO.

Melucci, A. (1985) 'The Symbolic Challenge of Contemporary Movements', *Social Research*, **52**(4): 789–816.

MHAC (1995) *The Mental Health Act Commission, Sixth Biennial Report 1993–95*. London, HMSO.

Milewa, T. (1997) 'Community Participation and Health Care Priorities: Reflections on Policy, Theatre and Reality in Britain', *Health Promotion International*, **12**(2): 161–8.

Miller, E.J. and Gwynne, G.V. (1972) *A Life Apart*. London, Tavistock.

Millett, K. (1991) *The Loony Bin Trip*. London, Virago.

MIND (1986) *Finding Our Own Solutions. Women's Experiences of Mental Health Care*. London, MIND.

MIND (1992) *Stress on Women. Policy Paper on Women and Mental Health*. London, MIND.

MIND (1997) *MIND Annual Review. Respect*. London, MIND.

Moodley, P. (1995) 'Reaching Out', in Fernando, S. (ed.) *Mental Health in a Multi-ethnic Society: A Multi-disciplinary Handbook*. London, Routledge.

Morris, J. (ed.) (1989) *Able Lives. Women's Experience of Paralysis*. London, Women's Press.

Mullender, A. (1991) 'Nottingham Advocacy Group: Giving a Voice to the Users of Mental Health Services', *Practice*, **5**(1): 5–12.

Nazroo, J. (1997) *Ethnicity and Mental Health*. London, Policy Studies Institute.

Nellis, M. (1999) 'Creating Community Justice', in Pease, K., Ballantine, S. and McLaren, V. (eds) *Crime Prevention*. London, IPPP.

Nelson, G. (1994) 'The Development of a Mental Health Coalition: A Case Study', *American Journal of Community Psychology*, **22**(2): 229–55.

Newman, J. and Clarke, J. (1994) 'Going About Our Business? The Managerialisation of Public Services', in Clarke, J., Cochrane, A. and McLaughlin, E. (eds) *Managing Social Policy*. London, Sage.

NHSE (National Health Service Executive) (1994) *Guidelines on the Discharge of Mentally Disordered People and their Continuing Care in the Community*. HSG(94)27. London, DoH.

NHSE (National Health Service Executive) (1995) *Priorities and Planning: Guidance for the NHS: 1996/9*. London, DoH.

NHSE (National Health Service Executive) (1996) *NHS Psychotherapy Services in England: Review of Strategic Policy*. London, DoH.

NHSME (1992) *Local Voices. The Views of Local People in Purchasing for Health*. London, DoH.

Nilbert, D., Cooper, S. and Corssmaker, M. (1989) 'Assaults Against Residents of a Psychiatric Institution: Residents' History of Abuse', *Journal of Interpersonal Violence*, **4**(3): 342–9.

Noble, P. and Rodger, S. (1989) 'Violence by Psychiatric In-patients', *British Journal of Psychiatry*, **155**: 384–90.

Nocon, A. and Qureshi, H. (1996) *Outcomes of Community Care for Users and Carers*. Buckingham, Open University Press.

Norris, M. (1984) *Integration of Special Hospital Patients into the Community*. Aldershot, Gower.

Oakley, A. (1980) *Women Confined. Towards a Sociology of Childbirth*. Oxford, Martin Robertson.

Offe, C. (1984) *Contradictions of the Welfare State*. London, Hutchinson.

Oliver, M. (1990) *The Politics of Disablement*. Basingstoke, Macmillan.

Oliver, M. (1996) *Understanding Disability. From Theory to Practice*. Basingstoke, Macmillan.

Parsloe, P. (ed.) (1996) *Pathways to Empowerment*, Series: Social Work in a Changing World. Birmingham, Venture Press.

Perkins, R. (1999) 'Madness, Distress and the Language of Inclusion', *Open-Mind*, **98**: 6.

Perkins, R., Nadirshaw, Z., Copperman, J. and Andrews, C. (1996) (eds) *Women in Context: Good Practices in Mental Health Services for Women*. London, Good Practices in Mental Health.

Phillips, A. (1993) *Democracy and Difference*. Cambridge, Polity Press.

Phillips, A. (1995) *The Politics of Presence*. Oxford, Clarendon Press.

Pilgrim, D. (1997a) *Psychotherapy and Society*. London, Sage.

Pilgrim, D. (1997b) 'Some Reflections on "Quality" and "Mental Health"', *Journal of Mental Health*, **6**(6): 567–76.

Pilgrim, D. and Rogers, A. (1993) *A Sociology of Mental Illness*. Buckingham, Open University Press.

Pilgrim, D. and Rogers, A. (1999) *A Sociology of Mental Health and Illness*, 2nd edn., Buckingham, Open University Press.

Pilgrim, D. and Waldron, L. (1998) 'User Involvement in Mental Health Service Development: How Far Can It Go?', *Journal of Mental Health*, **7**(1): 95–104.

Pithouse, A. and Williamson, H. (eds) (1997) *Engaging the User in Welfare Services*. Birmingham, Venture Press.

Pollitt, C. (1990) *Managerialism and the Public Services*. Oxford, Basil Blackwell.

Potier, M. (1993) 'Giving Evidence: Women's Lives in Ashworth Maximum Security Hospital', *Feminism and Psychology*, **3**: 335–47.

Pound, A., Mills, M. and Cox, T. (1985) 'A Pilot Evaluation of Newpin, a Homevisiting and Befriending Scheme in South London', *Newsletter of the Association of Child Psychology and Psychiatry*, October.

Prior, L. (1993) *The Social Organisation of Mental Illness*. London, Sage.

Prior, P. (1999) *Gender and Mental Health*. Basingstoke, Macmillan.

Prior, S., Stewart, J. and Walsh, K. (1995) *Citizenship: Rights, Community and Participation*. London, Pitman.

Pugh, R. and Richards, M. (1996) 'Speaking Out: A Practical Approach to Empowerment', *Practice* **8**(2): 35–44.

Putnam, R. (1993) *Making Democracy Work*. Princeton, Princeton University Press.

Ramon, S. (ed.) (1991) *Beyond Community Care. Normalisation and Integration Work*. Basingstoke, Macmillan.

Ramon, S. and Sayce, L. (1993) 'Collective User Participation in Mental Health: Implications for Social Work Education and Training', *Issues in Social Work Education*, **13**(2): 53–70.

Ranson, S., Martin, J., McKeown, P., Nixon, J. and Mitchell, R. (1995) 'Citizenship for the Civil Society', paper presented to the ESRC Local Governance Workshop, Participation, Citizenship and New Management, University of Birmingham, 4/5 October.

Read, J. and Baker, S. (1996*) Not Just Sticks and Stones. A Survey of Stigma, Taboos and Discrimination Experienced by People with Mental Health Problems*. London, MIND.

Riessman, F. and Carroll, D. (1995) *Redefining Self-help: Policy and Practice*. San Francisco, Jossey-Bass.

Ritchie, J., Morrissey, C. and Ward, K. (1988) *Keeping in Touch with the Talking. The Community Care Needs of People with Mental Illness*. Birmingham, Community Care Special Action Project, Social and Community Planning Research.

Rogers, A. and Pilgrim, D. (1991) '"Pulling Down Churches": Accounting for the British Mental Health Users' Movement', *Sociology of Health and Illness*, **13**(2): 129–48.

Rogers, E.S., Chamberlin, J., Ellison, M.L. and Crean, T. (1997) 'A Consumer-constructed Scale to Measure Empowerment Among Users of Mental Health Services', *Psychiatric Services*, **48**: 1042–7.

Rogers, H. (1999) 'He who Pays the Piper Calls the Tune – a Consideration of Managment Issues of Voluntary and Not for Profit Agencies in the Contracting Process', *Social Services Research*, **3**: 29–35.

Romme, M. and Escher, S. (1993) *Accepting Voices*. London, MIND.

Rosenhall, D.L. (1973) 'On being Sane in Insane Places', *Science*, 179: 250–8.

Ross, C.A., Norton, G.R. and Wozney, K. (1989) 'Multiple Personality Disorder. An Analysis of 236 Cases', *Canadian Journal of Psychiatry*, **34**: 413–18.

Rowbotham, S. (1992) *Women in Movement. Feminism and Social Action*. New York, Routledge.

Rowlands, J. (1998) 'A Word of the Times, but What Does it Mean? Empowerment in the Discourse and Practice of Development', in Afshar, H. (ed.) *Women and Empowerment. Illustrations from the Third World.* Basingstoke, Macmillan.

Ryan, J. and Thomas, F. (1980) *The Politics of Mental Handicap*. Harmondsworth, Penguin.

Sashidharan, S.P. (1993) 'Afro-Caribbeans and Schizophrenia: The Ethnic Vulnerability Hypothesis Re-examined', *International Review of Psychiatry*, **5**: 129–44.

Sashidharan, S. and Francis, E. (1993) 'Epidemiology, Ethnicity and Schizophrenia', in Ahman, W.I.U. (ed.) *'Race' and Health in Contemporary Britain*. Buckingham: Open University Press.

Sassoon, M. and Lindow, V. (1995) 'Consulting and Empowering Black Mental Health System Users', in Fernando, S. (ed.) *Mental Health in a Multi-ethnic Society: A Multi-disciplinary Handbook*. London, Routledge.

Scott, A. (1990) *Ideology and the New Social Movements*. London, Unwin Hyman.

Segal, S.P., Silverman, C. and Temkin, T. (1993) 'Empowerment and Self-help Agency Practice for People with Mental Disabilities', *Social Work*, **38**(6): 705–12.

Seidler, V. (1994) *Unreasonable Men: Masculinity and Social Theory*. London, Routledge.

Seidman, S. (1998) *Contested Knowledge. Social Theory in the Postmodern Era*. Oxford, Blackwell.

Seligman, M.E. (1975) *Helplessness*. San Francisco, Freeman.

Shaikh, A. (1985) 'Cross-cultural Comparison: Psychiatric Admission of Asian and Indigenous Patients in Leicestershire', *International Journal of Social Psychiatry*, **31**(1): 3–11.

Shakespeare, T. (1993) 'Disabled People's Self-organisation: A New Social Movement?', *Disability Handicap and Society*, **8**(3): 249–64.

Shakespeare, T. (1998) 'Social Constructionism as a Political Strategy', in Velody, I. and Williams, R. (eds), ibid.

Sheldon, B. (1984) 'A Critical Appraisal of the Medical Model in Psychiatry', in Olsen, M.R. (ed.) *Social Work and Mental Health*. London, Tavistock.

Sheppard, M. (1990) *Mental Health: The Role of the Approved Social Worker.* Joint Unit for Social Services Research. University of Sheffield/Community Care.

Showalter, E. (1987) *The Female Malady. Women, Madness and English Culture 1830–1980*. London, Virago.

SHSA (1993) *Report of Committee of Inquiry into Death in Broadmoor Hospital of Orville Blackwood and Review of Two Other Afro-Caribbean Patients (Big, Black and Dangerous)*. London, Special Hospitals Service Authority.

Sibley, D. (1995) *Geographies of Exclusion*. London, Routledge.

Simpson, T. (1995) 'Being Angry, Being Heard', *Open Mind*, **75**.

Skellington, R. and Morris, P. (1996) *'Race' in Britain Today*, London, Sage.

Social Services Committee (House of Commons) (1990) *Community Care: Choice for Service Users*, 6th Report. London, HMSO.

Soni Raleigh, V. and Balarajan, R. (1992) 'Suicide and Self-burning Among Indians and West Indians in England and Wales', *British Journal of Psychiatry*, **161**: 365–8.

Stallard, P. (1996) 'The Role and Use of Consumer Satisfaction Surveys in Mental Health Services', *Journal of Mental Health*, **5**(4): 333–48.

Sturdy, C. (1987) 'Questioning the Sphinx: An Experience of Working in a Women's Organisation', in Ernst, S. and Maguire, M. (eds) *Living with the Sphinx: Papers from the Women's Therapy Centre*. London, Virago.

Tarrow, S. (1998) *Power in Movement. Social Movements and Contentious Politics*. Cambridge, Cambridge University Press.

Taylor, M. (1992) *User Empowerment in Community Care: Unravelling the Issues*. Bristol, SAUS.

Taylor, P. and Gunn, J. (1999) 'Homicides by People with Mental Illness: Myth and Reality', *British Journal of Psychiatry*, **174**: 9–14.

The Avon Mental Health Measure (n.d) Bristol Social Services/South West MIND.

Thesen, J. (1997) *Brukermedvirkning i psykiatriske helsetjenester – Egenorganisering og andre organiseringsinitiative i Norge og England*. Conference report, University of Bergen, Norway, May.

Toffler, A. (1980) *The Third Wave*. New York, Morrow.

Took, M. (n.d.) *Mental Illness and the Services People Need. A Handbook for Professionals, Volunteers, People with a Mental Illness and their Family Carers*. Southampton, National Schizophrenia Fellowship.

Touraine, A. (1985) 'An Introduction to the Study of Social Movements', *Social Research*, **52**(4): 749–87.

Trainor, J., Shepherd, M., Boydell, K.M., Leff, A. and Crawford, E. (1997) 'Beyond the Service Paradigm: The Impact and Implications of Consumer/Survivor Initiatives', *Psychiatric Rehabilitation Journal*, **21**(2): 132–40.

Tudor, K. (1996) *Mental Health Promotion. Pardigms and Practice*. London, Routledge.

Turner, B.S. (1995) *Medical Power and Social Knowledge*. London, Sage.

Valentine, M.B. and Capponi, P. (1989) 'Mental Health Consumer Participation on Boards and Committees: Barriers and Strategies,' *Canada's Mental Health*, **37**(June): 8–12.

Van der Male, R. (1996) 'Users, Family Members and Professionals: Three Interests, One Goal'. Paper given to the 5th Congress of the World Association for Psychosocial Rehabilitation. Rotterdam, April.

Van Os, J., Castle, D.J., Takei, N., Der, G. and Murray, R.M. (1996) 'Psychotic Illness in Ethnic Minorities: Clarification from the 1991 Census', *Psychological Medicine*, **26**: 203–8.

Van Steenbergen, B. (ed.) (1994) *The Condition of Citizenship*. London, Sage.

Vandergang, A.J. (1996) 'Consumer/Survivor Participation in the Operation of Community Mental Health Agencies and Programs in Metro Toronto: Input or Impact?', *Canadian Journal of Community Mental Health*, **15**(2): 153–70.

Velody, I. and Williams, R. (eds) (1998) *The Politics of Constructionism*. London, Sage.

Wadsworth, Y. and Epstein, M. (1998) 'Building in Dialogue Between Consumers and Staff in Acute Mental Health Services', *Systemic Practice and Action Research*, **11**(4): 353–79.

Wainwright, H. (1994) *Arguments for a New Left. Answering the Free Marker Right*. Oxford, Blackwell.

Wallcraft, J. (1996) 'Some Models of Asylum and Help in Times of Crisis', in Tomlinson, D. and Carrier, J. (eds) *Asylum in the Community*. London, Routledge.

Warner, R. (1994) *Recovery from Schizophrenia, Psychiatry and Political Economy*. London, Routledge.

Watkins, T.R. and Callicutt, J.W. (1997) 'Self-help and Advocacy Groups in Mental Health', in Watkins, T.R. and Callicutt, J.W. *et al.* (eds) *Mental Health Policy and Practice Today*. Thousand Oaks, CA, Sage.

Westwood, S. *et al.* (1989) *Sadness in my Heart: Racism and Mental Health*. Leicester, Black Mental Health Group.

Wilkinson, R. (1996) *Unealthy Societies: The Afflictions of Inequality*. London, Routledge.

Wilkinson, S. and Kitzinger, C. (1994) 'Towards a Feminist Approach to Breast Cancer', in Wilkinson, S. and Kitzinger, C. (eds) *Women and Health. Feminist Perspectives*. London, Taylor and Francis.

Williams, J. and Lindley, P. (1996) 'Working with Mental Health Service Users to Change Mental Health Services', *Journal of Community and Applied Social Psychology*, **6**(1): 1–14.

Williams, J., Watson, G., Smith, H., Copperman, J. and Wood, D. (1993) *Purchasing Effective Mental Health Services for Women: A Framework for Action.* Canterbury, University of Kent.

Wilson, G. (ed.) (1995) *Community Care. Asking the Users.* London, Chapman & Hall.

Wilson, M. and Francis, J. (1997) *Raised Voices.* London, MIND.

Wilson, S. (1996) 'Consumer Empowerment in the Mental Health Field', *Canadian Journal of Community Mental Health*, **15**(2): 69–85.

Wolfensberger, W. (1972) *The Principle of Normalisation.* Canada, National Institute of Mental Retardation.

Wong, M.L. and Ku, K. (1996) 'Chinese Women', in Perkins, R., Nadirshaw, Z., Copperman, J. and Andrews, C. (eds) *Women in Context: Good Practices in Mental Health Services for Women.* London, Good Practices in Mental Health.

Wood, D. and Copperman, J. (1996) 'Sexual Harassment and Assault in Psychiatric Services', in Perkins, R., Nadirshaw, Z., Copperman, J. and Andrews, C. (eds) *Women in Context: Good Practices in Mental Health Services for Women.* London, Good Practices in Mental Health.

Wootton, B. (1958) *Daddy Knows Best.* Twentieth Century.

Young, I.M. (1996) 'Communication and the Other: Beyond Deliberative Democracy', in Benhabib, S. (ed.) *Democracy and Difference: Contesting the Boundaries of the Political.* Princeton, NJ, Princeton University Press.

Index

Page numbers in **bold**
represent major sections of
the text

A

abuse
  and experience of distress
    141
  psychiatric hospitals 11,
    74
  in public 16
  women 7, 74, 76–7, 79
  see also harassment;
    violence
academic issues 51, 55
  see also education;
    research and
    measurement
accountability 20, 50, 159
action and activists **47–56**
  autonomous, *see* autonomy
  black people 91–2
  collective, *see* collective
    action
  community 48
  direct 50, 145
  failure to act 4
  power of 21
  priorities 46
  single-issues 136
  social 134, 136–8
  users and workers 54
  voluntary, *see* voluntary
    action/organisations
  women 76–80
  see also campaigns and
    campaigning;
    empowerment and
    disempowerment;
    Health Action Zones;
    involvement strategies;
    movements
administrators and officials
    60–1, 101, 105, 112–14
  see also management
    issues; service staff
advocacy 8, 34–40
  black people 93
  community care White
    Paper 45
  empowerment 23
  misunderstanding of 129
  needs assessment 58

Norway 65
  self-advocacy 38, 40, 45,
    108, 133
  self-help groups 105,
    107, 110
  v. service provision 64
  UK Advocacy Network
    39–40, 48, 54–5
  women 36
  see also Nottingham
    Advocacy Group
African-Caribbean people
    36, 80–6, 88, 92
  see also black people
Afro-Caribbean Mental
  Health Project, Brixton,
  London 93
agency 15, 21, 70–2
  see also action and
    activists
aggression, *see* violence
Alcoholics Anonymous 108
Alleged Lunatics' Friends
  Society 27
All Wales Strategy for
  Mental Illness 102, 120
America, *see* North
  America; USA
anger 100
Angstringen 65
anti-depressants 83
anti-psychiatry 31–2
anxiety 158, 165
apathy 103
Approved Social Worker
  training 51, 129
arts 15, 50, 144, 147
  see also literature
Ashworth Hospital 36
Asians 81–5, 90, 92, 93, 158
  see also ethnic issues
assertive outreach 13
asylums 11, 26–9, 118, 155
  see also hospitals
attachment theory 72
attitudes
  professional **113–16**, 123,
    132
  public, *see* public opinion
Australia 12, 53
autonomy 95, **105–8**, **123–4**
  and citizenship 13–15

concept/definition of 7–9,
    16
  mental illness v. physical
    illness 12
  and MIND 38
  new social movements
    146, 150–2
  and participation 150–1
  service organisations 34
  see also self-help
Avon Mental Health
  Measure 58
Awaaz 93

B

Bangladeshis 81–2, 84
Barham, P. 6, 11, 17
Barnes, M. 12, 24, 57, 58,
    77, 105, 137, 140, 154
  and Barham, P. 6
  and Bowl, R. 80, 82, 88
  and Maple, N. 5, 71, 77,
    148
  and Prior, D. 56, 157, 160
  and Shardlow, P. 13, 96,
    105, 109–10, 124, 140
  and Stephenson, P. 77
  and Walker, A. 23
  and Warren, L. 18
  and Wistow, G. 54, 57, 59
  et al. (1990) 71, 87, 129
  et al. (1996) 49, 78
  et al. (1998) 46
  et al. (1999) 53, 59,
    60–1, 100
behaviour variations 5–6
  in consultation exercises
    100–1
  cultural 8, 86–7, 90
    see also ethnic issues
  gender issues 69–71
  sexual 71–2
  violent, *see* violence
Birmingham, UK 36, 43–4,
    51, 79, 156
Black Carers and Clients
  Project 93
black people **80–93**
  empowerment 141
  Health Action Zone
    programmes 158
  MPs 145
  needs of 163

182

perceived as dangerous
87–9
racism 7, 30
women 76, 140
see also African-Caribbean
people; Asians; ethnic
issues; Indians
Black Report 156
Blackwood, O. 88, 92
Blair, T. 157
Bottomley, V. 55
Bowl, R. 57, 125, 127,
129, 131, 165
and Barnes, M. 80, 82, 88
and Ross, K. 42, 97, 101,
103, 121, 123
Bradford Health Action
Zone 159
Brandon, D. 26, 31, 34, 125
Brighton Health Authority
37
Bristol Crisis Service for
Women 79
Brixton, London 93
Broadmoor High Security
Hospital 36, 92
Building Bridges 45, 113
Bureau of Community
Mental Health, Wisconsin
113–14
Busfield, J. 8, 27, 70, 73

C
Camberwell, London 73
campaigns and campaigning
50, 121
Campaign Against
Psychiatric Oppression
(CAPO) 54
civil liberties 32
ethnic minorities 90, 93
joint working 112
MIND 15, 37, 52
National Schizophrenia
Fellowship 39
priority given to 40
proactive 148
psychiatric hospitals 39,
42
public awareness 158
RESPECT 37
Stress on Women 37, 52,
77
voting rights 15
welfare benefits 66
What's going Wrong? 39
women's issues 76
see also action and
activists; lobbies

Canada 163
alternative services 123
consultation over
legislation 21
consumer organisations
63, 106
involvement initiatives
44, 102, 117
joint working 112
partnership 121
self-help tradition 64,
106, 108
women and abuse 74
see also Ontario; Toronto
cannabis 86
capacity and competence
3–9, 109
care
community, *see*
community care
continuity of 13
v. control in psychiatry 10
hospital, *see* hospitals
needs-led 57
primary 118
residential 97, 116
see also institutions
see also mental health
services; treatment issues
Care Programme Approach
procedures 120
carers
black people 93
community care policy
45, 57–8
empowerment of 23–4
health authority/social
service forums 120
lobby groups 131–2
National Schizophrenia
Fellowship 38, 47–8,
132
as partners in care 62
v. patients/users 23, 42,
120, 163
Carers' Recognition and
Services Act 1996 57
*Caring for People:
Community Care into
the New Decade and
Beyond* 44
Carroll, D. 106, 107 108,
114
Central Association for
Mental Welfare 28
Central Council for
Education and Training in
Social Work (CCETSW)
114

Chamberlin, J. 4, 64, 147
change 24, 30
barriers to 164
of diagnosis 86
environmental 97
individual lives/minds
94–116
in knowledge domain 67
limitations of **130–1**
in MIND 36
perceptions of 99, 104,
113–16, 132
see also public opinion
political 97
priorities for 66, 95
professionals **113–16**
resistance to 115–16,
124–7
rhetoric of 131
slow process 132
social 75, 97, **134–52**
social security 17
system 56, **117–33**
see also transformation
charitable sector, *see*
voluntary action/
organisations
Child Guidance Council 28
children 24, 34, 79
see also young people
Chinese Mental Health
Association 52
choice and choice-making
21, 57, 66, 109, 166
see also decision-making
Church, K. 21, 44, 100,
112, 115, 122, 163
citizenship **13–16**, 32, 66,
109, 149
civil rights, *see* rights issues
Clare, J. 26
class issues, *see* social class
clientenbond 34
clients 19, 42
see also service users
clinicians, *see* doctors;
medical profession
coalitions 44, 112, 121–2,
133
see also partnership
collective action/
organisations 15–16,
48–50
historical issues 27
and individual difference
68
new social movements
136, 146, 148
self-advocacy 108

women 72, 75–6
colour, *see* ethnic issues
Committee of Inquiry into
    Farleigh Hospital (1971)
    30
committee skills/structures
    100, 104, 124–7
Common Concerns
    conference (1988) 37
communication issues 87,
    92, 97, 101, 136
    see also terminology and
        discourse
communitarianism 160
community **156–62**
    action/development 48
    justice 161–2
    membership, *see*
        citizenship
    notion of 11–12
    safety 159–61
    supervision, *see*
        Community Treatment
        and Supervision Orders
    see also ethnic issues
community care
✓ v. asylums 11
    compulsion, *see*
        Community Treatment
        and Supervision Orders
    consultation on 57–8, 99
    Health Action Zones 62,
        158–9
✓ legislation 12, 14
    see also NHS and
        Community Care Act
    policy context 11–13, 45,
        56–8, 61–2
    psychiatric nurses 113
    residential care 97, 116
    resource shifting 122
? ──────White Paper 44–5
Community Mental Health
    Programme, Birmingham
    University 51
Community Mental Health
    Promotion 159–60
Community Organisation
    for Psychiatric
    Emergencies 34
Community Support
    Program (NIMH) 33
Community Treatment and
    Supervision Orders
    12–14, 38, 42, 55–6, 143
competence and capacity
    3–9, 109
compromise 148

compulsory detainment in
    hospital
    and autonomy 8
    black people 82, 87, 92
    and citizenship 14–15
    and power of professionals
        20, 30, 106
    social worker input 129
    study of 156
    women 71
    see also Mental Health Act
        of England and Wales
compulsory supervision/
    treatment, *see* Community
    Treatment and
    Supervision Orders
confusion 6, 97, 103, 105,
    116
consciousness-raising 75,
    108, 133, 135, 146
    see also public opinion
Conservative government
    35, 156
consultation **96–105**, **118–20**
    community care plans
        57–8, 99
    emotional exchange 115
    empowerment 21, 100,
        105
    v. participation 43
    policy making 55
    purpose of 96–8, 104
    success and failure of 130
    as therapy 104
    see also decision-making
consumers
    advocacy groups 23
    community care policy 57
    empowerment 58–9, 66–7
    families as 38
    in North America 2–3, 23,
        32–4, 43, 63, 106, 110
    satisfaction surveys 119
    terminology 2–3, 105
    and user movement
        emergence 139
    voice of 50
Consumer/Survivor
    Development Initiatives
    (CSDI) 65, 106–7
control issues
    v. care/desire to help
        10–11, 129–30
    over consultation 101
    empowerment/enabling
        19–24, 54, 130
    gender 78
    over health 24
    lack of 6, 7

legislation 162
management 127
professional 9–10, 49, 54,
    64, 98, 128, 131
self-help groups 107, 109
shared 128
social policy 10, 12, 129,
    140
welfare state 18
see also power
coping strategies 85, 109,
    117
counselling 118, 144
Court of Protection 14
creative therapies 144
crime/criminality 69–70,
    161
cultural issues
    action on mental health 52
    behaviour variations 8,
        86–7, 90
    belief systems 89–90
    cross-cultural studies 82,
        89
    new social movements
        135–8, 144–5, 147
    organisational 100
    self-help groups 107
    user movement 144
    see also arts; ethnic issues

D
Davey, B. 1, 23, 52, 143–4
day centres 83, 97, 122
decision-making **53**, **163–4**
    carers 48
    and consultation processes
        101–3
    health care v. social care
        58
    purchasing services 122
    resource distribution 20
    shared 20–1, 61
    staff selection 125–6
    user committees 98–9
    see also choice and
        choice-making;
        consultation;
        participation
definitions, *see* terminology
    and discourse
de-institutionalism, *see*
    institutions
delirium 10
dementia 5
democratic issues 34, 48,
    96–7
Department of Health
    Caring for People 44

Changing Childbirth 76
framework for mental
    health services 55
Health of the Nation 45,
    119
*Modernising Mental
    Health Services* 12, 61–2
Saving Lives 157–8
supervision registers 12
Working in Partnership
    45, 113–14
depression 73, 81–3, 86–7,
    108, 158
deprivation 84, 158
detainment, *see* compulsory
    detainment in hospital
diagnosis and misdiagnosis
    86–90
    ethnicity 80–1, 84, 87,
        92–3
    gender 76–7
    inconsistency 31, 86
    professional power 60
    psychiatric 3, 31, 33, 75
    schizophrenia 93
    stigmatising **16–17**, 49,
        110, 139–42
difference and diversity
    68–93
    in empowerment
        objectives/strategies 46,
        63–6, 130
    in involvement strategies
        35, 114
    in new social movements
        136, 141
    tolerance of 160
    types of user 33, 127, 163
    in user movement 48, 56,
        140, 154
    value of 141, 145
    see also ethnic issues;
        gender issues; otherness
disabled people/disability
    citizenship 149
    financial exchange 63
    medical model of 2,
        63–4, 146, 157–8
    new social movement 47,
        63, 66, 135, 137–8,
        141–2, 146
    social model of 146
    voluntary action 47
    welfare benefits 66
    women 76
discourse, *see* terminology
    and discourse
discrimination 37, 75, 84,
    110

see also race and racism
disempowerment, *see*
    empowerment and
    disempowerment
distress, mental/
    psychological, *see*
    psychological distress
diversity, *see* difference and
    diversity
doctors 59–60, 83, 118, 124
    see also medical
        profession/medicine
Doyal, L. 7–8, 75, 150–1
Dutch influences, *see*
    Netherlands

E

East London and City
    Health Authority 158
East Sussex Social Services
    department 37
eating disorders/distress
    49, 79
Economic and Social
    Research Council 156
economic issues 10–11,
    157–9
    rights, *see* rights issues
    see also socio-economic
        issues
Ecoworks, Nottingham 1,
    52, 144, 160
ECT 29, 83
education and training 49,
    164–5
    anti-racist 91, 93
    Health Action Zone
        programmes 158–60
    primary care staff 118
    self-help groups 107, 110
    skills 103–4, 107–9, 159
    social work 51, 113–14,
        129, 164
    in staff selection
        procedures 126
    users in **50–2**, 104, 113
electric shock treatment
    (ECT) 29, 83
Ely Hospital 31
emotional issues 144
    ethnic minorities 87
    in families 5–6
    normative assumptions
        141
    as source of knowledge
        128
    user consultation 115
    see also psychological
        distress

employment, *see* work
empowerment and
    disempowerment **1–25**,
    46–93
    autonomous action 105–6
    black people 141
    carers v. users 23–4
    citizen v. consumer 58–9,
        66–7
    in civil society 152
    complexity of notion 5,
        166
    concepts/definitions of 2,
        17–25, 66–7, 153
    and consultation exercises
        21, 100, 105
    and control 19–24, 54,
        130
    and difference/diversity
        68–93, 130
    future prospects **153–6**
    Health Action Zone
        policies 159
    and health inequalities 24
    as intervention technique
        96–7
    and knowledge 155
    measuring 18, 49
    multiple dimensions of 1,
        7
    objectives 46, **63–6**
    participation as
        disempowering 162
    partnership 20–1, 46,
        160, 166
    personal 49
    policy issues 9, 18, 49,
        67, 159
    political issues 18, 49,
        50, 97
    proactive/reactive 23
    self-help groups 109
    v. service provision 65
    social change 134
    as transformation 24, 67
    user committees 98
    users v. carers 23
    women 141
    see also involvement
        strategies; power
Enlightenment 27, 137
environmental issues
    v. biological model of
        medicine 27, 157–8
    ethnic minorities 84
    influenced by user
        involvement 97
    and mental health 143–4

new social movements
135, 137, 143
user-friendly
environments 102
see also social
circumstances/conditions
Epstein, M. 53, 127, 128–9
ethnic issues 68–9, 78,
80–93
action on mental health 52
banishment of 90
health inequalities 158–9
migration/selection
hypothesis 85
new social movements
135, 145
social exclusion 90, 161
women 76, 82, 84, 90,
93, 140, 158
see also black people;
cultural issues; race and
racism
Europe
civil rights 32
participatory democracy
26
social policy 153
women's experience 77
see also Germany;
Netherlands; Norway
European Court 15
European Regional Council
of the World Federation of
Mental Health 77
evaluation issues 57–8,
94–6, 104
see also research and
measurement
Everett, B. 108, 114, 116,
117, 118
exclusion, *see* social
exclusion/rejection
expenditure, *see* funding

F
families
as 'consumer lobby' 38
impact on 3, 5–6
source of tension 23
Tory policy 57
and women 76
Family Health Services
Authority 118
Farleigh Hospital 30, 31
fear 6, 89, 101, 129, 132
feedback 58, 60, 99, 103
females, *see* women
feminism 72, 75–6, 137,
138, 149

Fernando, S. 9, 84, 87, 88,
89
Figert, A. 10, 72, 77, 138
financial issues, *see*
economic issues; funding;
poverty
focus groups 58, **118–20**
folly 10
Forty Second Street,
Manchester 48
Foucault, M. 9–10, 22, 90,
138, 152
Fourth National Survey of
Ethnic Minorities 81
Frame, J. 29
freedom 14, 32
Friends of St Anne's
Orchard 54
frustration 105
funding 133
Consumer/Survivor
Development Initiatives,
Ontario 65–6, 106
priorities 131
from statutory
organisations 53
self-help groups 108,
110–11
voluntary organisations 63
see also resources
future prospects **153–66**

G
gay people 135, 137, 138,
142, 161
see also lesbians
gender issues 5, 8, **68–78**,
82, 149, 158, 163
see also men; women
general practitioners (GPs)
83, 118, 124
genetic factors 85
Germany 55
Good Practices in Mental
Health for Women 52,
77, 124
Gostin, L. 32, 129
Gough, I. 7–8, 150–1
government, *see* legal
system and legislative
issues; policy issues;
political issues
Graham Report 115
groups
advocacy 23, 34–40, 105
see also Nottingham
Advocacy Group
autonomous 105
see also autonomy

black 91
see also ethnic issues
consumer 23, 105, 122,
164
focus 58, **118–20**
interest 105
lobby 131–2
marginalised 138–9, 149,
159
see also social exclusion
pressure 105, 145
self-help/support 33, 39,
64–5, **105–11**, 133
skills in working with
103–4, 108–9
*see also names of
individual groups and
organisations*
Grow 64

H
harassment 16, 78, 161
Harding, S. 52, 137, 149
Harrison, G. 81, 86, 88
healing traditions 93
health
and empowerment 24
mental, *see* mental health
and illness
and social care practice,
see professionals and
professional practice
and social care system,
see welfare state/system
Health Action Zones
(HAZs) 62, 156–60
health authorities 37, 44,
63, 99, 120, 143, 158
health care market 62
Health Improvement
Programmes (HImps) 157
health inequalities 24,
76–7, 132, **156–62**
(The) Health of the Nation
45
health profesionals, *see*
professionals and
professionals practice
health status 157
health variations 156–7
see also health
inequalities
Hearing Voices
movement/network 48,
50
helper-therapy principle
108–11
Hieronymous, Bergen 65

historical issues **26–45**
  ethnic minorities and
    psychiatry 88
  inequalities 156
  managing madness 9–13
  self-help 105
  user movement 26, 35,
    139, 154, 166
holism 28, 144, 165
Holland 34–7, 55
hospitals
  abuse 11, 74
  admission rates **80–2**, 111
  black people 83
  campaign to keep open
    39, 42
  compulsory detention, *see*
    compulsory detainment
    in hospital
  discharge 12–13
  length of stay 111
  locked wards 83, 88
  long-stay 11–12
  patient advocacy/councils
    34, 36
  scandals 31
  secure/special 36, 77, 82,
    83
  see also asylums;
    institutions; treatment
    issues; *names of
    individual hospitals*
housing 16, 99, 107, 116,
  121–2
*How to Involve Users and
  Carers* 39
hysteria 70

I
identity 132, **140–3**
  ethnic 135, 145
  new social movements
    135–8, 146
  personal sense of 3–6, 9,
    14, 96
  shared 140
  women 72
  and work 136
  see also stigmatisation
ideological contexts 56, 87
Ignatieff, M. 5
illness, *see* mental health
  and illness
incompetence 7
Indians 81
individuals and
  individualism **94–116**
  autonomy 146, 152
  citizenship 15

and collective action 68
  Tory policy 57
  treatment issues 27
  see also personal
    experience/impact
inequality 24, 76–7, 132,
  156–62
Insane Liberation Front 33
insanity, *see* madness
insight 7, 20
institutions
  academic 51, 55
  institutionalism 11,
    117–18
  psychiatric 11
    see also asylums;
    hospitals
  racism 83, 149
  welfare, *see* welfare
    state/system
insurance companies 16
international issues 48, 124
  see also Canada; Europe;
    USA
interpersonal relationships
  3–9, 72
interventions, *see* treatment
  issues
intimidation 161
involvement strategies
  42–5, **94–7**, **165–6**
  black people 91
    see also ethnic issues
  differing perceptions 35,
    114
  disbenefit of 103
  as distraction 112
  goals of 96–8, 162
  as good practice 117
  grafted onto existing
    structures 131
  legislation 44–5, 57, 113,
    115, 117
  limited achievements of
    130
  models/opportunities for
    104
  North American 44, 102,
    113–14, 117
  policy making 51, 55,
    104, 114, 117
  research 94, 104–5, 118
  see also consultation;
    decision-making;
    empowerment and
    disempowerment;
    participation;
    partnership
irrationality **3–9**

J
jargon 99
  see also terminology and
    discourse
jobs, *see* work
joint working 44, 49, 99,
  112–13
justice and injustice 13, 69,
  145
*Justice Unbalanced:
  Gender, Psychiatry and
  Judicial Decisions* 69

K
Knowing Our Own Minds
  survey 51, 144
knowledge
  dissemination/production
    52, 67, 137–8
  emotional v. intellectual
    128
  growth in self-help groups
    109
  recognition of value in
    empowerment 155
  sharing 51
  subversive power of 22,
    67
  user 60, 104, 113–14,
    144, 165
  see also science

L
Labour government/
  movement 46, 134,
  156–7, 161
language, *see* terminology
  and discourse
learned helplessness 31
learning difficulties 24
legal rights, *see* rights issues
legal system and legislative
  issues **131–3**
  Canada 21
  community care/
    supervised discharge
    12, 14
    see also NHS and
      Community Care Act
  involvement strategies
    44–5, 57, 113, 115, 117
  non-compliance with
    medication 55
  preventive control 162
  service/treatment
    compulsion 143
    see also Community
      Treatment and
      Supervision Orders

terminology and discourse 69
Leicester Black Mental Health Group 91
Leonard Cheshire Foundation 47
lesbians 52, 76, 135, 137, 142
Lindow, V. 90, 91, 92, 93
literature and poetry 5, 29, 40, 50, 147
lobbies 38, 40, 131–2, 136, 145
    see also campaigns and campaigning
local authorities 61, 63, 99, 120
long-stay hospitals, *see* hospitals
(The) Loony Bin Trip 142
Lord, J. 44, 100, 102, 130
lunatics **26–45**
    see also madness; mental patients

M
MadNation 141
madness **9–13**
    fear of 6
    is feminine 69
    living with 4
        see also personal experience/impact
    'mad pride' 141
    as 'other' 90
    and sanity 141–3
    and science 9, 27–8
    terminology 3, 10
    and violence in media 140
    see also mental health and illness
Madness and Civilisation 9–10
magistrates 87
Major, J. 57, 156
males, *see* men
management issues
    hegemony 131
    madness **9–13**
    managerial imperative 42
    power of managers 59–61
    surveillance of professionals 127
    users on management committees 121
    see also administrators and officials; policy issues; professionals and professional practice

Manchester
    Awaaz 93
    Forty Second Street 48
Maple, N. 5, 71, 77, 148
marital status 5
market factors 62
mass media, *see* media
McCabe, S. 113, 114, 126
McLean, A. 2, 33, 43, 46, 63–5, 96, 110–11, 117, 132
McMurphy's, Sheffield 40–1, 64
measurement issues, *see* research and measurement
media
    black people 92
    campaigning 50
    questioning services 30
    resistance from local communities 116
    stereotypes 15
    stigmatisation 49
    television programmes 40
    violence 140
medical model of disability/illness 2, 63–4, 146, 157–8
medical profession/medicine
    biological focus 27–8, 85, 88, 132
    experimental research paradigm 118
    hegemonic control 9–10, 131
    see also doctors; nurses; professionals and professional practice; psychiatrists
medical treatment/medication, *see* treatment issues
melancholy 10, 27
Melucci, A. 135, 136, 146
men
    gay 135, 137, 138, 142, 161
    marital status 5
    suicide among young men 78
    see also gender issues
Mental Aftercare Association (MACA) 36
mental disorder 3, 7, 70–2, 142
    eating disorders 49, 79
    personality disorders 161
    psychosis 5, 55, 81–3, 86

    see also madness; mental health and illness; psychiatry; schizophrenia
mental distress, *see* psychological distress
Mental Health Act of England and Wales 3, 30
    community supervision/treatment 12
    compulsory detainment/'sectioning' 8, 14, 71, 87, 156
mental health and illness
    action on, *see* action and activists
    'cure' 6–7, 111
    as defined by Mental Health Act, *see* mental disorder
    diagnosing, *see* diagnosis and misdiagnosis
    distress of, *see* psychological distress
    education on, *see* education and training
    and empowerment, *see* empowerment and disempowerment
    and the environment, *see* environmental issues
    ethnicity, *see* ethnic issues
    experience of, *see* personal experience/impact
    gendered construction of, *see* gender issues
    holistic perspective 144, 165
    legislation, *see* legal system and legislative issues
    managers, *see* management issues
    medical model of 2, 63–4, 146, 157–8
    of NHS workforce 67
    nursing review (1994) 45, 113
    passivity in 17, 70–1, 75, 80
    patients, *see* mental patients
    v. physical illness 12
    policy on, *see* policy issues
    professionals in, *see* professionals and professional practice
    promotion of 160

radical analysis of 32
recovery 6–7, 111
services, *see* mental health services
social factors in, *see* social circumstances/conditions
staff, *see* service staff
terminology of, *see* terminology and discourse
treatment of, *see* hospitals; treatment issues
users, *see* service users; user movement
vulnerability factors 73–4, 83–4
women and, *see* women
workers, *see* professionals and professional practice; service staff
see also madness; psychiatry
Mental Health Foundation 51, 144
mental health services
access to 76, 102
alternative 15, 40, 49, 63, 77, 79, 123, 166
contracts 49, 63, 112
control over 23
see also control issues
delivering 113, 115
and dependency 33, 109
for ethnic minorities, *see* ethnic issues
evaluation of 57–8, **94–6**, 104, 113, 115
see also research and measurement
experience of receiving 3, 85
see also personal experience/impact
inappropriate 85
mainstream 79, 104, 121, 124, 144
managing, *see* management issues
monitoring 57–8, **94–6**, 104, 113, 115
out-patient 82
planning 99, 102, 113, 115, 119, 121
protective role of 4, 10–14, 78
providers/purchasers 63, 99, 122, 131
response to distress 85
self-referred 83

shaping public perceptions 67
for women 74
see also care; National Health Service; service organisations; service staff; service users
Mental Health Services Consumer Group, Newcastle 122, 164
Mental Health Social Work Award 114
Mental Health Task Force 55
mental hospitals, *see* hospitals
mental hygiene movement 28, 118
mental illness, *see* mental health and illness
mental patients
advocacy for, *see* advocacy
autonomy of, *see* autonomy
as citizens **13–16**, 32, 66, 109, 149
dangerous 69–70, 161
see also violence
detained, *see* compulsory detainment in hospital
discharge from long-stay hospitals 12–14
ethnic minorities, *see* ethnic issues
ex-patients 2, 63–4, 75
see also survivors
lunatics **26–45**
see also historical issues
patient councils 34, 36, 39, 121
Patient's Charter 154
power over, *see* power
racism, *see* race and racism
record as 7
safety of, *see* safety issues
supervision of 12–14, 38, 42, 55–6
and supporters, *see* carers
as victims 17, 161
voice of 29, 36, 50, 79, 102, 156
as whole persons 28, 144, 165
see also mental health and illness; service users
Mental Patients Union 34
Merseyside 66

methodology, *see* research and measurement
Millett, K. 3–4, 77, 142
MIND
advocacy v. service provision 64
campaigns 15, 37, 52
Common Concerns conference (1988) 37
local associations 36
membership 37–8
Nottingham 36
Open Mind 141
RESPECT campaign 37
Solihull 51, 68
stigma survey 16
voting rights campaign 15
Women In Mind 77
World Federation of Mental Health conference (1985) 37
see also National Association for Mental Health
MINDLINK 37, 47, 55
misdiagnosis, *see* diagnosis and misdiagnosis
Modernising Mental Health Services 12, 61–2
mood swings 5
moral issues 11, 28
Morris, J. 58, 76, 138
movements
asylum 118
civil rights 30, 32
consumer 32
de-institutionalisation 118
disability 47, 63, 66, 135, 137, 138, 141–2, 146
environmental 135, 137, 143
ethnic identity 135, 145
ex-patients 75
feminist 137
gay/lesbian 135, 137, 142
hearing voices 50
identity v. interest-based 137, 138
labour 134
mental hygiene 28, 118
new, *see* social movements
patch 41
peace 134, 137
self-help 64
social 30, 105, 117, 132, **134–52**
solidarity in 93, 152
success of 133

survivor/user, *see* user
   movement
women's 30, 75–6, 134,
   135, 140
youth 134
mutual aid 109–11
   see also self-help

N

National Alliance for the
   Mentally Ill 33
National Alliance of Mental
   Patients 33
National Alliance of
   Psychiatric Survivors 33
National Association for
   Mental Health (NAMH)
   30, 32
   see also MIND
National Association of
   Patients Councils 34
National Campaign for
   Civil Liberties 32
National Council for Mental
   Hygiene 28
National Foundation of
   Patient Advocates 34
National Health Service
   (NHS) 29, 61, 156
   NHS and Community
   Care Act 1990 44,
   56–7, 63, 113
   NHS Executive 12, 144
National Health Service
   Management Executive 44
National Institute of Mental
   Health Community
   Support Program 33
national issues 48–9, 55,
   124
   see also welfare state/
   system
National Mental Health
   Consumers Association 33
National Schizophrenia
   Fellowship (NSF) 38–9,
   47, 132
Nazroo, J. 5, 81, 83, 84,
   85, 86
needs
   assessment 58
   black people 163
   definition of 3
   needs-led care 57
   professional judgement on
   29
   special needs 31
   universal 150–1
   user views on 95, 109

negotiation skills 103
Nelson, G. 112, 121, 122,
   133
Netherlands 34–7, 55
neurosis 5
Newcastle 122, 164
New Labour government
   46, 156–7, 161
NEWPIN 78–9
New Zealand 115
NHS and Community Care
   Act 1990 44, 56–7, 63,
   113
NHS Executive 12
normalisation 31, 140–2,
   150
North America 64, 153
   see also Canada; USA
Norway 55, 65, 147
Nottingham Advocacy
   Group (NAG) 35–6, 156
   conference which founded
   UKAN 39
   and Ecoworks 1, 52, 144,
   160
   and participation 100, 164
   patient advocacy 124
   public awareness
   campaigns 158
   and Purchasing for Users
   Group (PUG) 122
   and service provision 64
Nottingham Health
   Authority 143
Nottingham Patients Council
   Support Group 39
Nottingham Purchasing for
   Users Group (PUG) 122,
   164
nurses
   mental health nursing
   review (1994) 45, 113
   professional power 60
   psychiatric 10, 113, 129

O

officials, *see* administrators
   and officials
older people 159
Oliver, M. 13, 32, 138,
   141, 145, 146
*One Flew Over the
   Cuckoo's Nest* 40
Ontario 65, 101, 106, 112,
   115, 121
Open Mind 141
oppression 7, **53–6**, 74, 91,
   136, 138

Orville Blackwood Inquiry
   88
otherness 90, 132, 141
outcome measures 58
outreach, assertive 13

P

parents, *see* families
Parsloe, P. 18–19, 22–3
Pathways to Empowerment
   18–19, 22–3
participation 42–5,
   96–102, 162–3
   and autonomy 150–1
   black people 91–2
   blurring of boundaries 48
   v. consultation 43
   democracy 26
   differing perceptions of
   35
   disempowering 162
   facilitating 164
   as goal in itself 97, 130
   Health Action Zone
   policies 159
   Nottingham Advisory
   Group 100, 164
   v. partnership 44
   political 136
   purpose of 96–8
   self-help groups 110
   and social change 145
   in society 95
   stress of 103
   success and failure of 130
   women 75
   see also decision-making
partnership 113, 115,
   121–2
   carers 62
   empowerment 20–1,
   45–6, 160, 166
   equal 164
   Health Action Zone
   policies 159
   joint working 112
   v. participation 44
   policy context 61–2
   social workers 129
   terminology 46
   in training 165
   voluntary organisations
   61–2, 163
paternalism 18, 30, 38, 60
patients, *see* mental patients
Perkins, R. 77, 124, 141,
   142

personal experience/impact **3–9**, **94–6**, 141–2, 147
defining and naming 2, 155
depersonalising practice 30–1
differences in 68
empowerment 49
ethnicity 83–4, 87, 91
historical 26–7, 29
interpersonal relationships **3–9**, 72
sense of self 3–6, 9, 14, 96
shared 140
and wisdom 107
see also individuals and individualism
personality disorders 161
philanthropy 28
Phillips, A. 136, 137, 145
physical abuse, *see* abuse
physical threat, *see* violence
Pilgrim, D. 10
and Rogers, A. 26, 34, 38, 54, 86, 88, 90, 105, 139, 140, 147
and Waldron, L. 102, 120, 164
poetry 5, 29, 40, 50, 147
police 61, 87, 161
policy issues **56–63**, **131–3**
anti-racist 91, 93
community care 11–13, 45, 56–8, 61–2
consultation on 55
control 10, 12, 129, 140
day centres 97
deinstitutionalism 11
empowerment 9, 18, 49, 67, 159
Health Action Zones 62, 156–60
health inequalities 157
new social movements 137, 150
North America 153
rights, *see* rights issues
segregation 11–12
targets for improvement 119
user involvement 51, 55, 104, 114, 117
political issues
Conservative government 35, 156
diagnostic process 87
empowerment 18, 49, 50, 97
identity 136

New Labour government 46, 156–7, 161
new social movements 133–9, 144–6
pluralism 137, 146
and schizophrenia 10
see also action and activists; campaigns and campaigning
(The) Politics of Disablement 32
(The) Politics of Mental Health 32
poverty **16–17**, 63, 66, 159
power
authority 20
balance of 43, 154, 156
black people 92
coercive 20–1
see also Community Treatment and Supervision Orders; compulsory detainment in hospital
consultation exercises 100
decision-making 21
delegated 20
and dominant discourse 138, 152, 160
electric shock treatment 29
ethnicity and gender 68
generative 21
legislative 14
loss of, *see* powerlessness
managers 59–61
patriarchal 75
professional 9–10, 19, 30, 42, 55, 57–60
relations 20, 75, 106, 109, 134, 160
resources 20, 112–13
sexual 74
sharing 43
subversive/through resistance 22, 67
transferred to users 42–3
welfare state 18
women 70–4
see also control issues; empowerment and disempowerment
powerlessness 20, 68, 70–2, 165
prejudice, *see* discrimination
pre-menstrual syndrome 10, 72
pressure groups 105, 145
primary care 118

see also community care; general practitioners
Prior, D. 56, 157, 160
private sector 61–3
probation service 61
problem-solving 20
see also decision-making
professionals and professional practice
allies or oppressors? **53–6**
see also partnership
changing attitudes **113–16**, 123, 132
collaboration or conflict with 53–6
see also consultation; participation
control by, *see* control issues
decision-making 20
dehumanising/depersonalising 30–1
discourse 69, **127–30**
disputes 10
education of, *see* education and training
expectations of **130–1**
as experts 27–8, 50, 60–1, 107, 132
good practice 77, 117, 124
green 52
joint working 44, 49, 99, **112–13**
v. managers 59–60
members of MIND 38
needs assessment 29
peer reviewed standards 59
power of, *see* power
range of 10
surveillance of activities 127
see also management issues
user knowledge 104, 113–14
see also involvement strategies; service users
in voluntary associations 28
women 77
see also doctors; medical profession/medicine; nurses; psychiatrists; service staff; social work/workers
'prosumers' 107
psychiatric diagnosis, *see* diagnosis and misdiagnosis

psychiatric disorder, *see* mental disorder
psychiatric hospitals, *see* hospitals
psychiatric interventions, *see* treatment issues
psychiatric nurses 10, 113, 129
psychiatric patients, *see* mental patients
psychiatric services, *see* mental health services
psychiatrists 10, 54–5, 86
psychiatry
  and abuse of women 74
  anti-psychiatry 31–2
  biological 74, 132
  confidence in 31
  cultural issues 82, 87–90
  diagnosis, *see* diagnosis and misdiagnosis
  discourse of, *see* terminology and discourse
  dominance of 129
  emergence of 27–8
  forensic 82
  and gender, *see* gender issues
  racism in 88
  see also ethnic issues
  role of 10
  and science 31
  and the welfare state **29–35**
  see also mental health and illness
psychoanalysts 10
psychological distress **3–9**
  affecting anyone 7, 68
  alternative explanations 50–1, 77
  demonisation of 132
  destructive impact of 4–5
  distribution of 68
  environmental circumstances 143
  see also social circumstances/ conditions
  ethnicity, *see* ethnic issues
  erratic/exhausting nature of 103
  experience of, *see* personal experience/impact
  gender differences, *see* gender issues
  incidence rates **80–2**, 84–6

normality of 140–1
ownership of 10
passivity 17, 70–1, 75, 80
prevalence of 73–4
reporting of 85
terminology of, *see* terminology and discourse
and work 10–11
see also emotional issues; mental health and illness
psychologists 10
psychosis 5, 55, 81–3, 86
  see also schizophrenia
psychotherapists 10
psychotropic drugs 71
public health 160–1
public opinion **113–16**
  barrier to community care 12
  changing 99, 104, **113–16**, 132, 158
  confidence in staff 29–30
  dangerousness of mental patients 161
  ethnic minorities 84, 87
  exclusionary 16
  self-help initiatives 108, 110
  shaped by mental health services 67
  Skeffington initiatives 33
  social movements 150
  see also consciousness-raising
public order/safety, *see* safety issues
public policy, *see* policy issues
Purchasing for Users Group (PUG), Nottingham 122, 164

Q
Quad 110–11

R
race and racism **86–93**
  and experience of distress 7, 30, 84, 141
  feminist theory 76
  institutional 83, 149
  'new' 90
  scientific 88
  women 140
  see also ethnic issues
radicalism 32, 34, 50
Rampton Special Hospital 36

random controlled trials 94–5
rationality and irrationality **3–9**
Recovery Incorporated 64
Reflect, Solihull 156
rejection, *see* social exclusion/rejection
relatives, *see* families
relativism 136
research and measurement
  barriers to change 164
  consultation exercises 119
  empowerment strategies/ values 18, 49
  ethnic issues 86
  evaluation 57–8, **94–6**, 104
  gender issues 72
  health inequalities 156
  involvement strategies 94, 104–5, 118
  joint working 112
  mental health of NHS workforce 67
  partnership 121
  paucity of 118, 139
  professional attitudes 115–16
  self-help groups 106
  by service users **50–2**
  see also surveys
residential care 97, 116
resistance 22, 93, 115–16, 124–7, 142
  see also campaigns and campaigning
resources
  community 122
  educational/training 51–2, 107
  power over 20, 112–13
  resource mobilisation theory 132–3
  and resistance 53
  staffing 131
  see also funding
Reville, D. 44, 112, 122
Riessman, F. 106, 107 108, 114
rights issues
  citizenship 13–15
  civil rights movement 30, 32
  definition of identity 146
  legal/procedural 110
  Patient's Charter 154
  reproductive rights 76
  women's rights 76

risk aversion 133
Rogers, A. 26, 34, 38, 54, 86, 88, 90, 105, 139, 140, 147
Ross, K. 42, 97, 101, 103, 121, 123
Royal College of Psychiatrists 12

S

safety issues 10–14, 42, 132–3
  black people 82
  community 159–61
  Health Action Zone programmes 159, 161
  women 77–8, 148
  see also compulsory detainment in hospital
Sainsbury Centre for Mental Health 51
sanity 141–3
Sashidharan, S. 80, 81, 85, 86, 112, 117
Sassoon, M. 90, 91, 92, 93
Saving Lives: Our Healthier Nation 157
scapegoats 90
Scar Tissue 5
schizophrenia
  ethnic issues 81, 86, 89, 90, 93
  National Schizophrenia Fellowship 38–9, 47, 132
  personal experiences 95
  and political economies 10
  redefining the experience 32
  socio-economic class 158
science
  v. emotional experience 128
  feminist 137
  and madness 9, 27–8
  and psychiatry 31
  racism 88
  recognition by users 54
  in USA 132
Scott, A. 137, 145, 146, 150, 152
screening 73
  see also research and measurement
sectioning, *see* compulsory detainment in hospital
Segal, S.P. 33, 64, 106, 108, 114
segregation 11–12

see also social exclusion/rejection
Seidman, S. 52, 136, 137, 142
self-advocacy 38, 40, 45, 108, 133
self-confidence 96, 104, 109
self-determination 33
self-efficacy 130
self-esteem 96, 109, 158–9
self-harm/injury 49, 79
self-help 33, 39, 64–5, **105–11**, 133
self-in-relation 72
self-interest **148–52**
self-perception 3–6, 9, 14, 96
  see also identity
self-referral 83
self-respect, *see* self-esteem
service contracts 49, 63, 112
service organisations
  autonomous 34
    see also autonomy
  collective, *see* collective action/organisations
  cultural issues 100
  decision-making **163–4**
  influence of user involvement 117
  mutual aid/self-help 33, 39, 64–5, **105–11**, 133
  separate/state-supported 53
  user-based, *see* involvement strategies; user movement
  voluntary, *see* voluntary action/organisations
  see also names of individual organisations and groups
service staff
  communication channels 97
  conflicting demands **127–30**
  ethnic minority 92–3
  primary care 118
  public confidence in 29–30
  racism 91
  resources for 131
  selection procedures 125–6, 155
  training, *see* education and training
  as users of services 67

see also administrators; professionals and professional practice
service users
  action, *see* action and activists
  black, *see* black people
  burn-out 103–4
  and carers 23, 42, 120, 163
  committees 97–100, 104, 121, 131, 162–3
  competing interests of 42
  consultation issues, *see* consultation
  councils 59–60
  as customers 57
    see also consumers
  discourse of, *see* terminology and discourse
  diversity of 127, 163
    see also difference and diversity
  education, *see* education and training
  ethnic minority, *see* ethnic issues
  excluded 43
    see also social exclusion/rejection
  expectations of **130–1**
  as experts 60, 114
  feedback from 58, 60, 99, 103
    see also involvement strategies
  following through their ideas **120–1**
  forums for 39, 99, 102, 105, 120–1
  individual, *see* individuals and individualism
  involvement in decision-making 53
    see also decision-making; involvement strategies
  joint working 44, 49, 99, **112–13**
  needs of, *see* needs
  organisation of, *see* user movement
  participation of, *see* participation
  partnership issues, *see* partnership
  patients, *see* mental patients

potential 43
power of, *see*
  empowerment and
  disempowerment
priorities 40, 46, 66, 95,
  99, 131
representation of 38,
  101–4, **124–7**, 163
research **50–2**
  see also research and
  measurement
responsibility of 57, 103,
  109, 148
role models 109
satisfaction surveys 58,
  119
self-help 33, 39, 64–5,
  105–11, 133
sites of action **47–56**
  see also action and
  activists
surveys of, *see* surveys
terminology, *see*
  terminology and
  discourse
as trainers **50–2**, 104, 113
  see also education and
  training
uncertainty about validity
  of opinions 102
views of 50, 118–19
  see also feedback
  see also survivors; user
  movement; women
sexism 149
  see also gender issues
sexual abuse, *see* abuse
sexuality
  female 71–2
  gay, *see* gay people
Shardlow, P. 13, 96, 105,
  109–10, 124, 140
Sheffield 40–1, 52, 64, 93
shell shock 28–9
Shifting the Balance plan,
  Birmingham 43–4
Skeffington initiatives 33
skills development/training
  103–4, 107–9, 159
Smythe, T. 32
social action 134, 136–8
  see also action and
  activists; movements
social change 75, 97,
  134–52
social class 76, 135–6, 158
social cohesion 157
social circumstances/
  conditions 17, 28, 74, 84

see also environmental
  issues; socio-economic
  issues
social constructionism 138
social control 10, 12, 129,
  140
social exclusion/rejection
  16–17
  civil rights 14
  communitarian
    perspectives 160–1
  disempowering impact 7
  ethnic minorities 90, 161
  fear of madness 6
  gays/lesbians 142, 161
  Health Action Zone policy
    157, 159
  marginalised groups
    138–9, 149, 159
  see also compulsory
    detainment in hospital;
    segregation
social history, *see* historical
  issues
social movements, *see*
  movements
social networks 49
social order 9
  see also safety issues
social policies, *see* policy
  issues
social relations 136, 142
social rights, *see* rights
  issues
social security issues 17
social services 60, 120
  departments 37, 44, 99,
    101
  see also welfare state/
    system
social theory 138
social work/workers
  empowerment 19
  managing madness 10
  Mental Health Social
    Work Award 114
  partnership study 129
  'patch' 41
  status of 60
  training 51, 113–14, 129,
    164
society
  citizenship 15
  contemporary 135
  empowerment 152
  participation in 95
  post-industrial/modern
    136
  protection of 10–12

role of people in distress
  10–11
values of 143
  see also state
socio-cultural factors, *see*
  cultural issues; ethnic
  issues
socio-economic issues 66,
  84, 157–60
  see also poverty; social
    circumstances/conditions
Solihull 51, 68, 156
Somalis 52, 93
special needs 31
spiritual aspects 144
stakeholders 19, 48, 61
state
  citizenship 15
  see also national issues;
    welfare state/system
stereotypes 15, 72, 80, 85,
  89, 155
stigmatisation **16–17**, 49,
  110, 139–42
strategies
  of black people 93
    see also ethnic issues
  coping 85, 109, 117
  for empowering users, *see*
    empowerment and
    disempowerment
  for involving users, *see*
    involvement strategies
  of social movements 148
    see also action and
    activists; campaigns and
    campaigning;
    movements
Strategies for Living
  programme 51, 144, 160
stress 84, 103, 159
Stress on Women
  (MINDLINK) 37, 52, 77
subversion 22, 67
suicide 78, 158
supervision, community/
  compulsory 12–14, 38,
  42, 55–6
support
  alternative models of 49,
    63, 77, 79
  black people 93
  community 33
  self-support 95
  stigma 16
  women 75, 77, 79
    see also self-help
surveys 41, 58, **118–20**, 144
  ethnic minorities 81

see also research and
measurement
survivors **26–45**, **138–40**
Consumer/Survivor
Development Initiatives
(CSDI) 65, 106–7
in North America 106
terminology 2–3, 40
see also service users
Survivors Speak Out (SSO)
39, 40, 48, 54–5
symptoms 31, 33, 95–6, 132

T
Task Force User Group 55
television programmes 40
see also media
terminology and discourse
2–3, **127–30**
autonomy 7–8
citizenship 13–14
community 11–12
consumers 2–3, 105
criminal justice 69
dominant discourses 22,
138, 152, 160
empowerment **17–24**
gays/lesbians 142
hysteria 70
legal 69
madness 3, 10
managerial 59
of meetings 126
mental disorder 7
new social movements
134, 136
partnership 46
poverty 17
professional 69, 129
psychiatric 17, 33, 69, 90
self-help groups 105
survivors 2–3, 40
see also communication
issues
Thatcher, M. 57, 156, 157
theatre 147
therapy, *see* treatment issues
'Third Way' 157
Toronto 104, 122
Tory government, *see*
Conservative government
training, *see* education and
training
Training and Enterprise
Councils (TECs) 61
Trainor, J. 46, 63–5, 107,
109, 111
tranquillisers 79, 83

transformation 24, 67,
135–6, 155
see also change
treatment issues **96–7**
alternative 51, 63, 124,
144
chemical suppresion of
symptoms 132
community 12–14, 38,
42, 55–6, 143
see also community care
complementary 51, 144
consent 14
consultation as 104
v. control/segregation
10–11
counselling 118, 144
creative therapies 144
electric shock 29, 83
ethnicity 68, 80, **82–3**,
85, 88–9, 92
fairness 13
gender 76, 73
'helper-therapy' **108–11**
iatrogenic effects 33
individualism 27
limited achievements of
31
non-compliance 55
prescribing as power 60
psychotropic drugs 71
restraining 89
talking 83, 144
therapeutic imperative 34
therapeutic relationships
19
women 148
trust building 104

U
UK Advocacy Network
(UKAN) 39–40, 48, 54–5
unemployment 16–17, 63,
84
Unzicker, R.E. 113, 114,
126
user movement **134–52**
black people in **90–3**
see also ethnic issues
development/evolution of
26, 35, 139, 154, 166
see also historical issues
diversity of **35–42**, 46,
48–50, 56
see also action and
activists; autonomy;
difference and
diversity; ethnic
issues; gender issues;

self-help; service
organisations
goals of 13, 46, **63–6**,
105, 135–6, 140, **165–6**
lack of research 118, 139
see also research and
measurement
oppositional nature of
112, 117, 148
radical 34, 50
and service provision 64,
148
summary of impact 124,
132
tensions in 38, 42, 129
vulnerability/weakness of
139, 147
women in 76
see also service users
USA
alternative services 123,
166
biological roots of distress
132
black people 91
civil rights 32
consumers 2–3, 23, 32–4,
43, 63, 106, 110
involvement strategies
113–14, 117
joint working 112
new social movements
137
partnership initiatives
121–2
practitioner goals 96
self-help tradition 64,
106, 111, 133
terminology 2
women's experience 74–6
User Voice, South
Birmingham 36, 79, 156

V
Victorian times 27–8, 90
see also historical issues
violence
black people 88–9
gender issues 70, 74
and madness in media 140
segregation policies 11
victims of 161
see also abuse
visual arts 15, 147
voice/s
expression of 29, 36, 50,
79, 102, 156
hearing 48, 50
women 145

Voices Forum/Network
(NSF) 38, 47, 54
voluntary action/
organisations **47–8**
advocacy v. service
provision 64
consultation issues 57–8
health authority/social
service forums 120
historical aspects 28, 30,
36, 39
lesbian women 52
partnership 61–2, 163
service level agreements
63
women-centred 78
*see also names of
individual organisations*
voting rights, *see* rights
issues

W
Wadsworth, Y. 53, 127,
128–9
Wainwright, H. 75, 138,
145
Waldron, L. 102, 120, 164
war 28–9
welfare professionals, *see*
professionals and
professional practice
welfare state/system **29–35**
benefits 66, 110
changes in 56, **117–33**
complexities of 16
crisis in 139
developments in
1970s–80s **41–5**
other countries than UK
65
pluralistic 61
power of 18
redistributive policies 157
see also social services
wellbeing 95, 109, 158–9
We're Not Mad We're Angry
40

We Shall Overcome,
Bergen 65
White Papers 12, 44–5,
157–8
white people 68
see also ethnic issues
Whittingham Hospital 31
Wisconsin Bureau of
Community Mental
Health 113–14
women **69–75**
abuse 7, 74, 76–7, 79
activism 72, **76–80**
advocacy groups 36
awareness 76
complex lives 77
compulsory detainment
71
connectedness 72
disabled 76
empowerment 141
ethnic minorities 76, 82,
84, 90, 93, 140, 158
Good Practices in Mental
Health 77, 124
lesbians 52, 76, 135, 137,
142
marital status 5
McMurphy's, Sheffield
40
MPs 145
organising **75–6**, 78
over-represented in mental
health system 73
passivity/powerlessness
70–5, 80
paternalism 30
pre-menstrual syndrome/
'raging hormones' 10,
72
refuges/safety of 77–8,
148
self-identification 72
sexual behaviour 71–2
Stress on Women
(MINDLINK) 37, 52, 77
support for 75, 77, 79

and therapists 74
voice for 145
vulnerability factors
73–4, 84
working class 140
see also feminism; gender
issues
Women In MIND 77
Women In Special
Hospitals and Secure
Units (WISH) 77
women's movement 30,
75–6, 134, 135, 140
Women's Space 78
Women's Therapy Centres
148
work
black people 84, 92
dismissal from 16
and experience of distress
10–11
Health Action Zone
programmes 158–9
and identity 136
joint working 44, 49, 99,
112–13
self-help groups 110
social, *see* social
work/workers
youth, *see* young people
Working in Partnership 45,
113–14
World Federation for
Mental Health
conferences (1985; 1995)
37, 40, 54–5
European Regional
Council 77

Y
young people 40, 48, 78,
134, 159
see also children

Z
Zito Trust 132